Contrast-Enhanced Ultrasound in Clinical Practice

Liver, Prostate, Pancreas, Kidney and Lymph Nodes

Contrast-Enhanced Ultrasound in Clinical Practice

Liver, Prostate, Pancreas, Kidney and Lymph Nodes

Thomas Albrecht
Lars Thorelius
Luigi Solbiati
Luca Cova
Ferdinand Frauscher

Preface by
Marcus Hörmann

Springer

Thomas Albrecht
Department of Radiology
and Nuclear Medicine
Berlin, Germany

Lars Thorelius
Department of Radiology
University Hospital Linköping
Linköping, Sweden

Luigi Solbiati
Luca Cova
Department of Radiology
General Hospital
Busto Arsizio, Varese, Italy

Ferdinand Frauscher
Department of Radiology II
University Hospital Innsbruck
Innsbruck, Austria

ISBN 88-470-0304-0 Springer Milan Berlin Heidelberg New York

Springer is a part of Springer Science+Business Media
springeronline.com

Printed in Italy

Cover design: Simona Colombo, Milan
Typesetting: Graficando, Milan
Printing and binding: Arti Grafiche Nidasio, Milan

Preface

The value of ultrasound contrast agents (USCA) in clinical practice depends on the pharmacokinetics, the signal processing, and the contrast-specific imaging modalities.

USCA are exogenous non-toxic substances smaller than red blood cells, which after intravenous administration must be stable enough to pass through the pulmonary capillary bed and enter the blood pool producing the necessary contrast enhancement for the duration of the examination. Recently, second-generation agents, such as SonoVue (Bracco Imaging SpA, Milan, Italy), have been introduced into the market. These agents, taking advantage of the stability of their microbubbles, withstand the acoustic pressure of insonation much better than previous USCA, resulting in an increased half-life of the agent and thus in a prolonged diagnostic window. These agents are blood pool agents that remain in the intravascular compartment and do not leak into the organ tissue. Therefore, they are used to increase the Doppler signal amplitude during their dynamic vascular phase. Concomitant with the improvement of contrast agents, different contrast-specific imaging modalities have been developed which, used in combination with USCA and a low mechanical index (MI), allow continuous real-time grey-scale imaging. These recent technical improvements have opened new possibilities in the use of USCA in a variety of indications, as shown in the contributions contained in this book. In the following chapters, some of the most distinguished users of second-generation USCA will share their knowledge and experience.

The first contributor is Dr. Thomas Albrecht, Department of Radiology, University Hospital of Berlin, Germany. Dr Albrecht discusses how to distinguish between benign and malignant focal liver lesions by evaluating various dynamic vascular patterns of the second-generation USCA.

Dr. Lars Thorelius of the Department of Radiology, University Hospital of Linköping, Sweden, explains the use of USCA in indications beyond the liver and shares his experience in diseases of the kidneys and pancreas.

The third contribution is from Dr. Luigi Solbiati, Department of Radiology, General Hospital of Busto Arsizio, Varese, Italy. Dr. Solbiati presents the preliminary results of the use of USCA in the characterization of reactive and malignant lymph nodes, with emphasis on the technical improvement of transducers.

Finally, Dr. Ferdinand Frauscher, Department of Radiology II, University Hospital Innsbruck, Austria, describes how the application of USCA is a promising and useful tool for the detection and clinical staging of prostate cancer.

In conclusion, this publication represents an overview of current and possible future new applications of USCA in routine and clinical practice by some very experienced experts.

Marcus Hörmann
Department of Radiology
University Hospital Vienna, Austria

Contents

Thomas Albrecht

Chapter 1

Dynamic Vascular Pattern of Focal Liver Lesions with Contrast-Enhanced Ultrasound: Latest Results with SonoVue

Thomas Albrecht
Department of Radiology and Nuclear Medicine
Berlin, Germany

Modern liver imaging of cancer patients requires an imaging modality that is not only highly sensitive in detecting lesions but also provides reliable characterisation of lesions and thus allows differentiation of metastases from frequently found benign lesions.

Conventional ultrasound (US) has a relatively poor sensitivity and specificity for imaging focal liver lesions, and US used to be inferior to CT and MRI mainly due to a lack of contrast agents. This has changed with the advent of microbubble contrast agents for US. The use of recent contrast agents such as SonoVue (Bracco Imaging SpA, Milan, Italy) combined with low-mechanical index contrast-specific imaging techniques such as Contrast Pulse Sequencing provides high-quality, dynamic, real-time imaging of focal liver lesions in the arterial, portal venous and delayed phase.

This improves lesion detection and characterisation. The typical dynamic features of all common focal liver lesions are discussed in this chapter and clinical results are presented.

Introduction

Both benign and malignant focal liver lesions are extremely common, and imaging the liver for focal lesions especially in cancer patients is one of the most frequent tasks in everyday radiological practice.

The most common malignancy of the liver are metastases from other organs: 25-50% patients with a known non-haematological malignancy have liver metastases at the time of diagnosis [1] with decreasing frequency in colon, gastric, pancreatic, breast and lung cancer [2]. The second most common malignant liver tumour is hepatocellular carcinoma (HCC). It is strongly associated with chronic viral hepatitis and cirrhosis and this is an important differential diagnostic clue. Other primary malignant liver tumours such as cholangiocarcinoma are much rarer.

The prevalence of solid benign liver tumours has been reported to be more than 20% in autopsy series [1, 3], and in patients with malignancy 25-50% of lesions under 2 cm in size are benign [4, 5]. The most frequent benign lesion is haemangioma with a prevalence of 7-21% [3, 6], followed by focal nodular hyperplasia (FNH), which has a prevalence of up to 3% [3, 7]. Adenomas are much rarer than FNH (by a factor of approximately 50) and they occur almost exclusively in female patients with a history of oestrogen medication. Other rare benign lesions are pyogenic, parasitic or fungal abscesses. Areas of focal fatty change or focal fatty sparing are very common; they do not represent true lesions but may appear as pseudo-tumours on ultrasound (US) and are thus easily confused with real tumours such as metastases. From the above it is obvious that imaging of focal liver lesions requires an imaging modality that is not only highly sensitive in detection but also provides reliable characterisation of lesions and thus allows differentiation of malignant from benign tumours. Characterisation of focal liver lesions by imaging is based on the assessment of the dynamic enhancement patterns of a focal liver lesion.

Contrast-enhanced US (CEUS) is a relatively new imaging technique that combines excellent contrast and spatial resolution with unrivalled temporal resolution of more than ten frames per second. CEUS is ideally suited for comprehensive dynamic real-time imaging of the contrast behaviour of focal liver lesions, especially if recent perfluor gas-based contrast agents such as SonoVue (Bracco SpA, Italy) combined with low-mechanical index (MI) contrast-specific imaging are used.

General Principles of Contrast-Enhanced Liver Sonography with SonoVue

CEUS of the liver and other abdominal organs requires contrast-specific imaging techniques. These techniques selectively display the non-linear response from contrast microbubbles with a high sensitivity. The most widespread contrast-specific mode is phase or pulse inversion harmonic imaging. It exploits mainly the second harmonic microbubble response.

SonoVue microbubbles consist of sulphur hexafluoride, which has a much lower water solubility than air and thus a higher bubble stability in the blood pool. SonoVue microbubbles are strong non-linear reflectors even at low MI, when only minimal microbubble destruction occurs. This means that they provide strong and continuous signal enhancement on low-MI CEUS, permitting continuous imaging of the liver for several minutes after injection.

In the liver, SonoVue is used for dynamic real-time imaging during the arterial (up to 30 s p.i.), portal venous (40 s–2 min p.i.) and delayed phases (>2 min p.i.). The delayed phase is a particular property of several US contrast agents, during which the microbubbles pool in the liver sinusoids; the precise reason for this phenomenon remains unclear. It begins approximately 2 min after injection and in case of SonoVue it persists for about 3 min. The delayed phase is particularly useful for characterisation of focal liver lesions since almost all malignant lesions (with the exception of some HCCs) are hypoenhancing in this phase, while the large majority of solid benign lesions show considerable delayed contrast uptake. Furthermore, the detection rate of malignant lesions and especially of metastases is highest on delayed-phase imaging. The delayed phase of SonoVue is fundamentally different from the "equilibrium phase" of non-specific contrast agents for CT and MRI. Instead, it is more comparable to delayed imaging with liver-specific agents for MRI.

Low-MI Real-Time Imaging with SonoVue: Examination Technique

Prior to contrast medium injection, a detailed unenhanced baseline examination of the liver is performed. This includes the use of tissue harmonic imaging and power Doppler to assess lesion vascularity. The baseline images are used to assess the hepatic anatomy and any masses, including cysts, typical haemangiomas and any solid masses which might be metastases. Baseline images are the basis for planning the contrast-enhanced scan, and the findings of both parts of the examination are interpreted together.

SonoVue is injected intravenously followed by a 10-ml normal saline flush. The typical dose is 2.4 ml; if necessary two further injections and/or a dose of 4.8 ml can be administered. It is mandatory to use contrast-specific imaging modes for post-contrast scanning. The acoustic output of the US system must be controlled carefully by the operator: best results are usually obtained at an MI of 0.1-0.2 and it should not exceed 0.3, as this would result in considerable bubble destruction and reduction of the contrast effect.

If solid lesions are already detected on the baseline scan, one or several of these will be selected for arterial phase imaging. The imaging plane should be selected in such a manner that as many lesions as possible are covered during the arterial phase. Sweeping through the liver during the arterial phase may be required to cover several lesions. This can be technically demanding, since the arterial phase lasts for only 10-15 s and more than one injection may be required. In most cases, however, it is sufficient to study one or two representative lesions in the arterial phase.

The portal venous phase (40 s to 2 min) and the delayed phase (2-5 min) last much longer, and the entire liver is continuously surveyed in multiple planes during these phases in a similar way as routine unenhanced scanning is performed. This will include lesions studied in the arterial phase, so that the enhancement patterns of these lesions can be assessed during all three phases.

For image documentation, representative digital movie clips of the relevant parts of the liver are recorded during all three phases. Alternatively, or in addition, still images can be obtained. Review of the recorded clips or of the cine loop after completion of the examination is often very helpful for comprehensive assessment of the liver without time constraints.

Dynamic Imaging Features of Metastases

Metastases show characteristic features in all three phases after contrast agent injection (Fig. 1). In the arterial phase the appearances are twofold: hypovascular metastases appear as hyporeflective lesions usually with a typical rim enhancement of varying size (Fig. 2A), while hypervascular metastatic deposits appear as brightly enhancing hyper-reflective and homogeneous lesions,

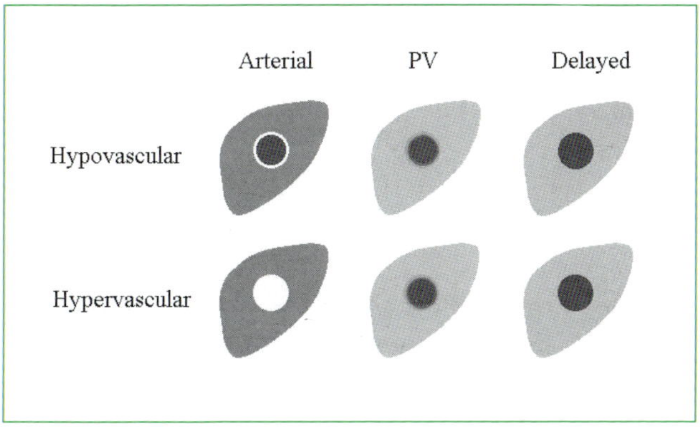

Fig. 1. Schematic display of the dynamic enhancement of hypo- and hypervascular metastases after SonoVue enhancement during the arterial, portal venous (PV) and delayed phase

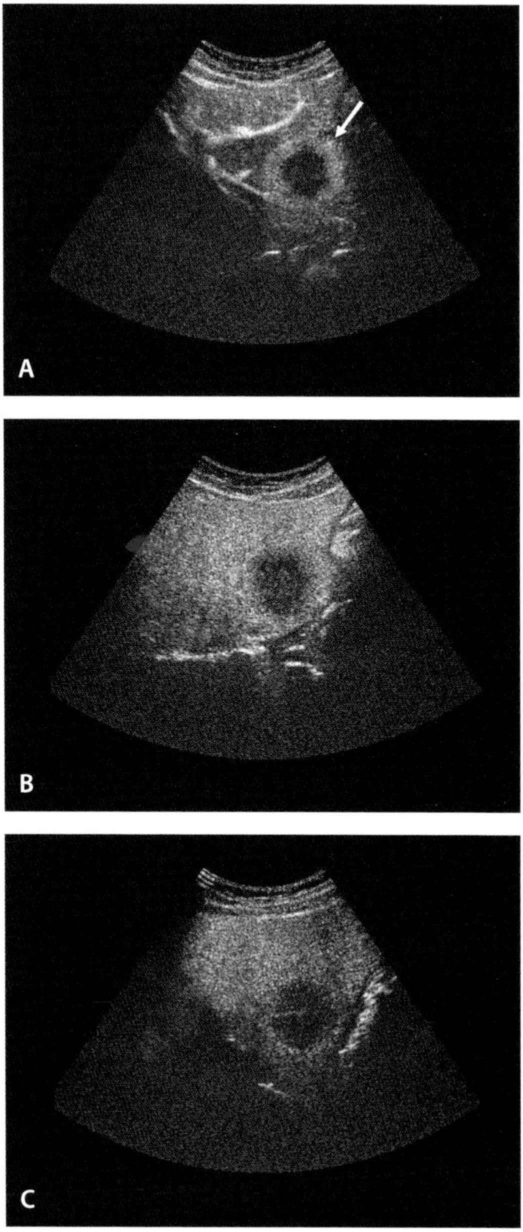

Fig. 2. "Hypovascular" hepatic metastasis from breast carcinoma. **A** In the arterial phase after SonoVue administration, the lesion displays strong peripheral rim enhancement (*arrow*). **B** Portal venous phase imaging shows fading of the rim. **C** In the delayed phase, the lesion presents as a hypoechoic enhancement defect with sharp margins

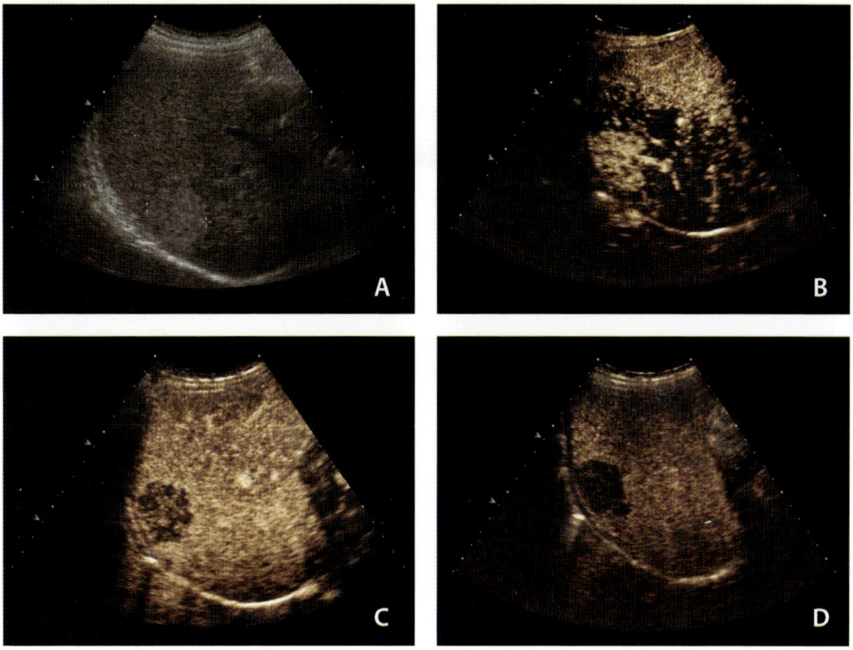

Fig. 3. Hypervascular metastasis. **A** Baseline grey-scale image with a slightly hyperechoic lesion. **B** During the arterial phase the lesion shows homogeneous enhancement while most of the liver parenchyma is only partially filled with contrast material. **C** Partial washout of contrast material from the lesion, which is now hypo-enhancing compared to homogeneously enhancing normal liver. **D** Complete washout of contrast material from the lesion in the delayed phase results in a sharply circumscribed "punched out" enhancement defect

sometimes with non-enhancing necrotic areas. At the beginning of the portal venous phase, the (rim) enhancement fades and the entire lesion becomes increasingly hyporeflective (Fig. 2B).

In the delayed phase, both hypo- and hypervascular metastases invariably appear as dark defects while the enhancement persists in normal liver parenchyma (Fig. 2C). During this phase the lesions are usually particularly well defined often with sharp, "punched out" borders. Both portal venous and delayed-phase imaging markedly increase the contrast between the enhancing normal liver and the non-enhancing metastases and thus improve detection, especially of small lesions less than 1 cm in diameter (Figs. 4, 5) and of lesions that are isoechoic on baseline.

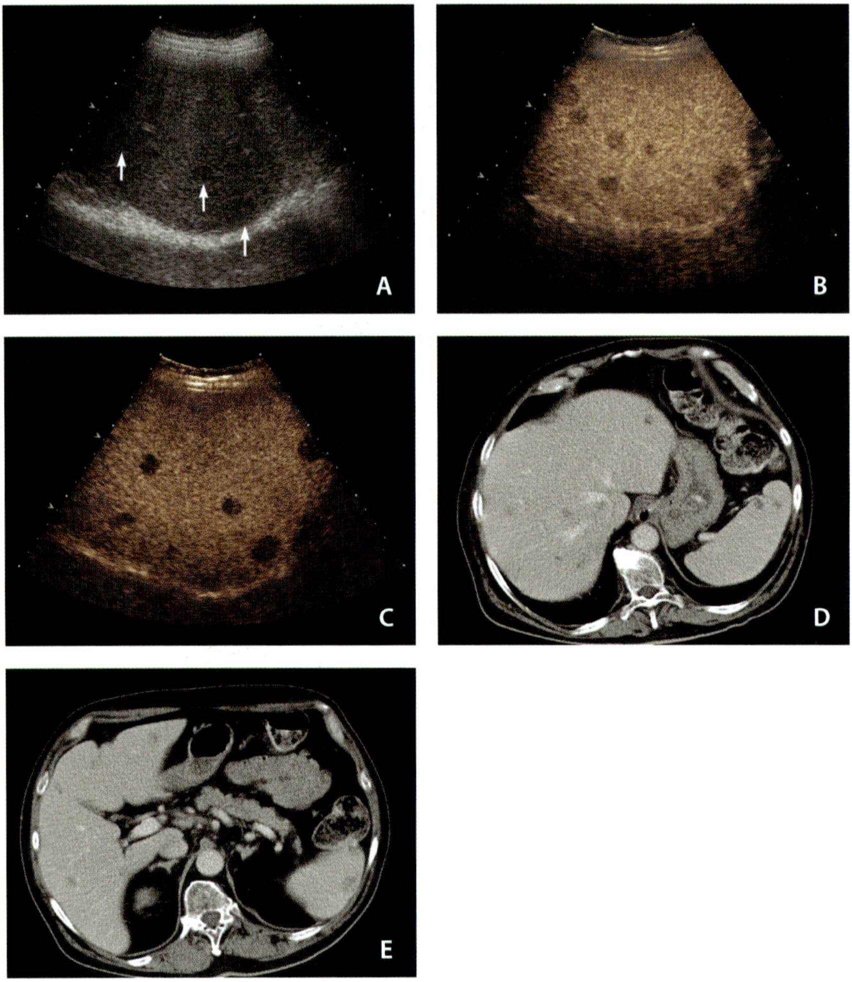

Fig. 4. Patient with multiple metastatic deposits. **A** Baseline US shows three ill-defined hypoechoic lesions in a slightly heterogeneous liver. **B, C** In the portal venous and delayed phase after SonoVue (Bracco Imaging, Italy) administration, multiple lesions are revealed throughout the liver, some of them only a few millimetres in diameter. **D, E** Multi-detector CT in the portal venous phase (150 ml Iohexol 300 Schering AG, Berlin, Germany) confirms the presence of multiple lesions

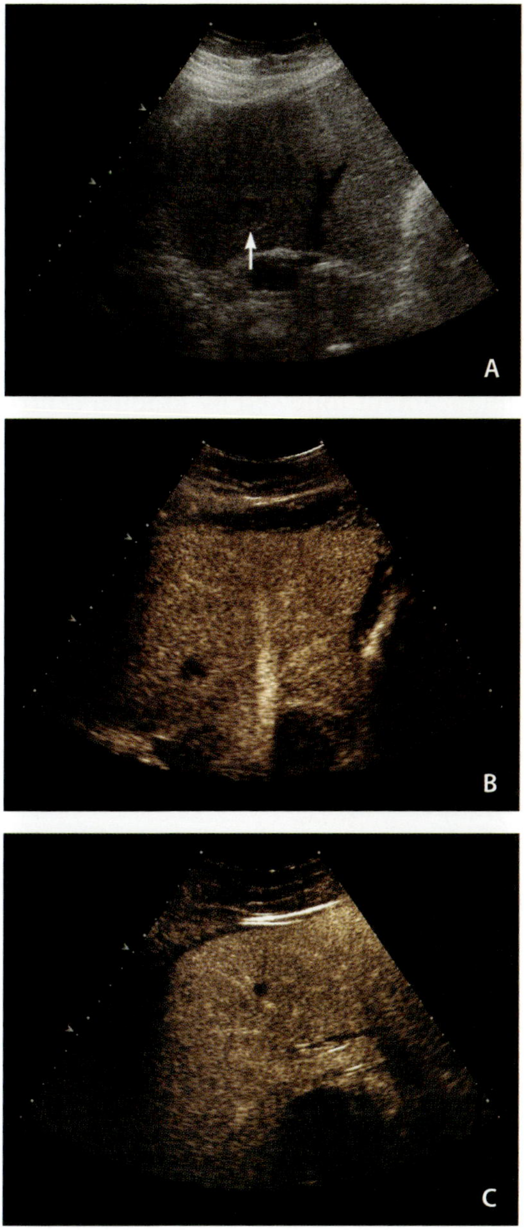

Fig. 5. Patient with bronchogenic carcinoma. **A** Baseline scan shows a single hypoechoic metastasis (*arrow*) in segment IV close to the left hepatic vein. **B** After administration of SonoVue (late phase), this lesion appears as a typical enhancement defect. **C** A second metastases of 6 mm is revealed after contrast administration (portal venous phase) in segment IV/VIII

Dynamic Features of Common Benign Lesions

As discussed above, solid benign liver lesions are very common. It is therefore of utmost importance to differentiate these from metastases in cancer patients. Fortunately, all common solid benign liver lesions have characteristic dynamic imaging features on CEUS and their diagnosis is thus usually unproblematic. Most of these features are analogous to those of dynamic CT and MRI.

Haemangiomas show a characteristic peripheral nodular arterial phase enhancement followed by gradual centripetal in-filling during the later phases (Figs. 6-8). The filling may be partial (Fig. 8) or complete. The speed of filling is size dependant: while small haemangiomas often fill within less than 1 min (Fig. 7), large lesions may take 5 min or more. Many large haemangiomas will not fill completely, but this can also occur in smaller lesions and can sometimes lead to confusion with metastases.

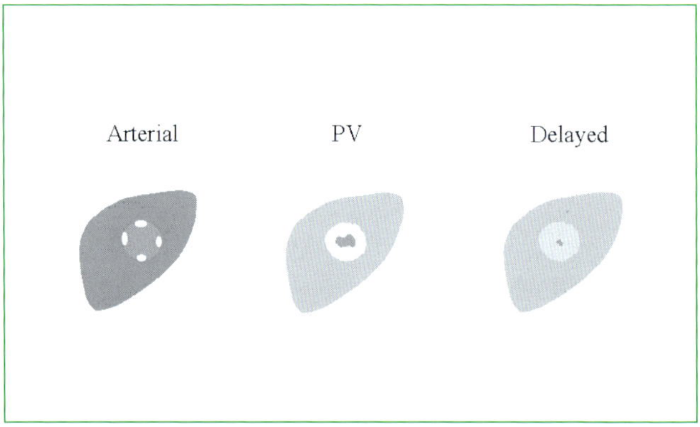

Fig. 6. Schematic display of the dynamic enhancement of haemangiomas after SonoVue administration during the arterial, portal venous (PV) and delayed phase

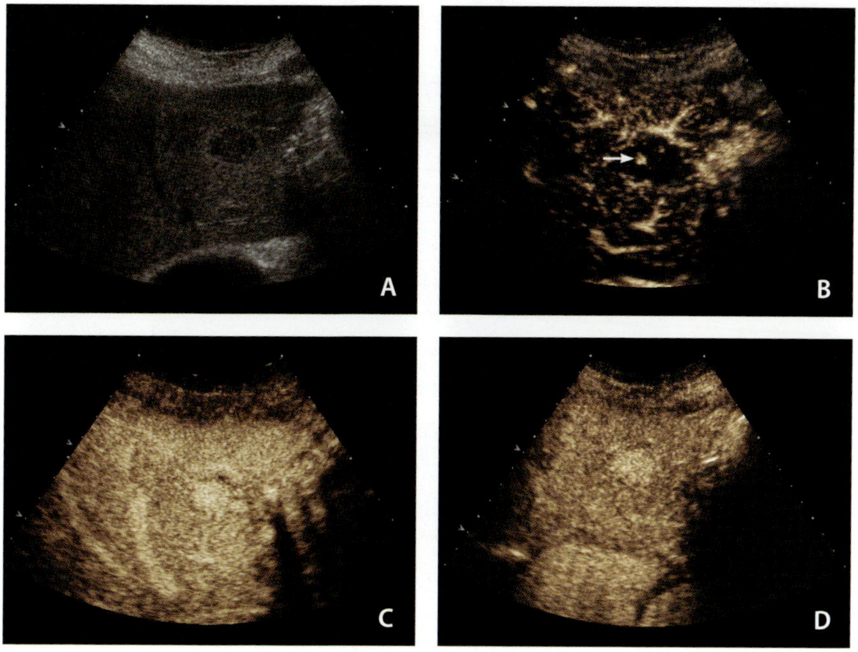

Fig. 7. Atypical haemangioma on conventional US with typical dynamic enhancement pattern after SonoVue administration. **A** Baseline US shows a 2-cm hypoechoic lesion in segment II, suggestive of a metastasis. **B** In the arterial phase, peripheral nodular enhancement is seen (*arrow*). **C, D** Complete filling of the lesion with microbubbles in the portal venous and delayed phase

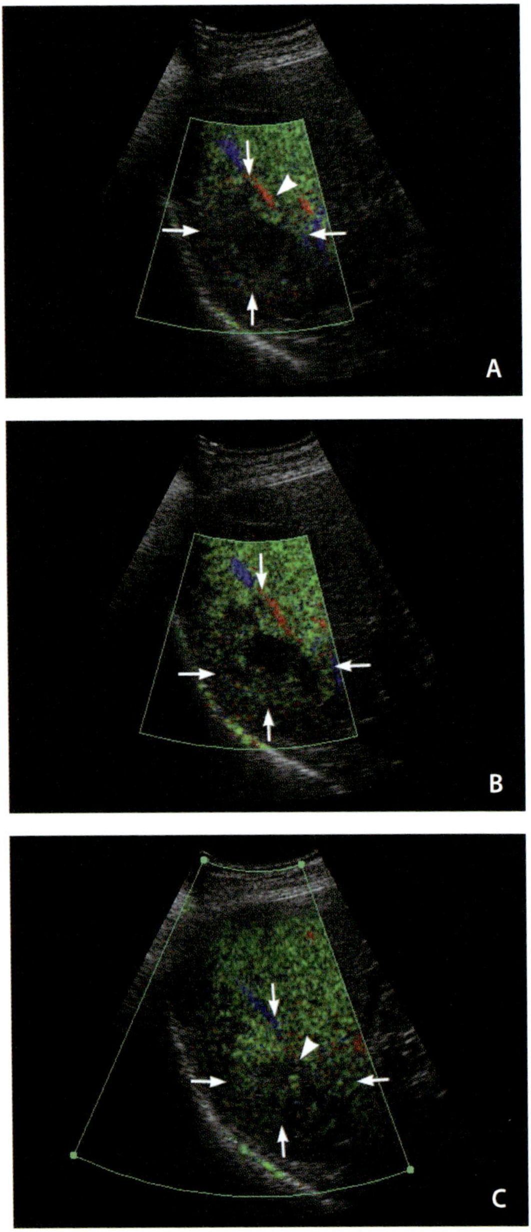

Fig. 8. Haemangioma (*arrows*). **A** Peripheral nodular enhancement (*arrowhead*) in the arterial phase. **B** In the portal venous phase the lesion shows some centripetal filling. **C** Most of the lesion has filled in the delayed phase with the exception of a small central area (*arrowhead*). Note: with this imaging technique (Vascular Recognition Imaging, VRI, Toshiba, Zoetermeer, The Netherlands), stationary microbubbles are displayed in green, flowing bubbles in red or blue

FNHs appear as lesions with homogeneous enhancement in the arterial phase. In about 50% of FNHs this is preceded by a typical spoke-wheel arterial pattern with centrifugal filling early in the arterial phase, lasting for a few seconds (Figs. 9, 10). In some cases the feeding artery is also seen (Fig. 11).

In the subsequent phases the lesions show a similar degree of enhancement as the normal liver, due to the liver-like tissue that the lesion consists of. Delayed-phase imaging is particularly useful for FNHs as they invariably appear as isoechoic or hyperechoic lesions, often with a non-enhancing central scar that was previously invisible (Figs. 9, 10). They are thus easily distinguished from metastases. Not unusually, especially when small, FNHs may disappear completely in the delayed phase due to their liver-like contrast behaviour.

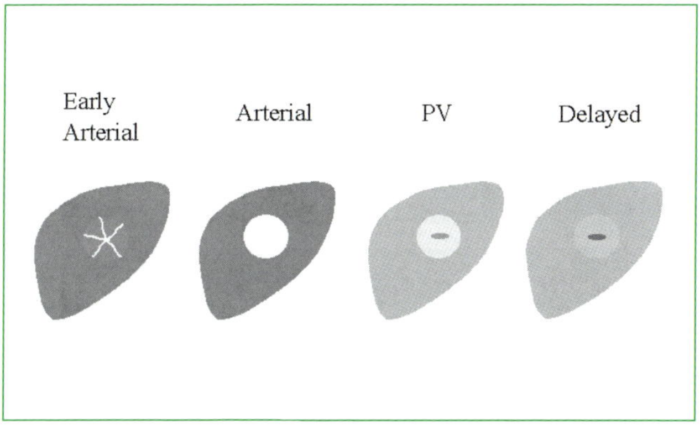

Fig. 9. Schematic display of the dynamic enhancement of FNH after SonoVue administration during the arterial, portal venous (PV) and delayed phase

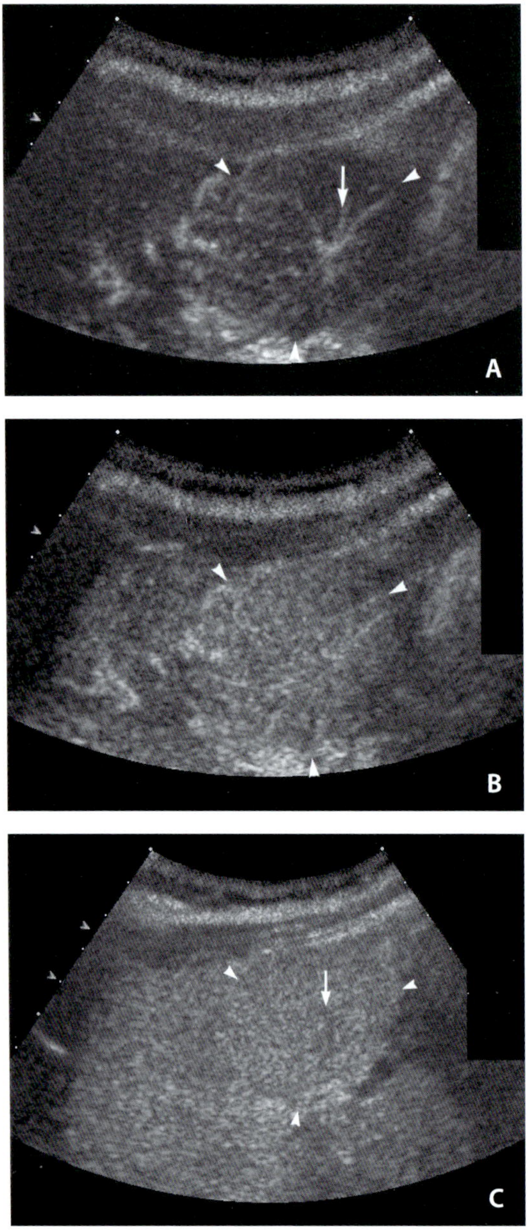

Fig. 10. Focal nodular hyperplasia (*arrowheads*) after SonoVue administration, imaged with phase inversion. **A** Typical spoke-wheel vascular pattern in the early arterial phase 13 s after SonoVue administration (*arrows*). **B** Three seconds later the lesion is completely filled with contrast material and appears hyperechoic to normal liver. **C** In the delayed phase the lesion is isoechoic to normal liver (*arrowheads*) with the exception of a small hypoechoic central scar (*arrow*)

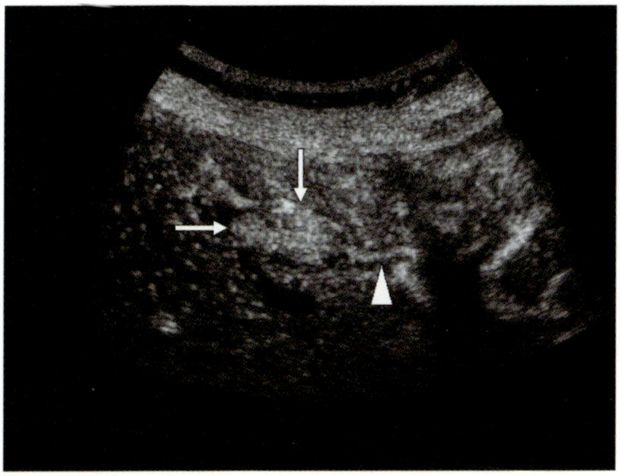

Fig. 11. Arterial phase of a FNH (*arrows*) showing strong homogeneous arterial enhancement and a typical feeding artery (*arrowhead*)

Focal fatty change and focal fatty sparing show the same contrast behaviour as normal liver parenchyma on all phases, since they contain no abnormal vessels and essentially consist of normal parenchyma. Again, these lesions usually "disappear" after contrast agent injection (Fig. 12).

Liver abscesses are uncommon in the western world they may, however, be confused with metastases since they also show a rim enhancement in the arterial phase and produce enhancement defects in the later phases. An important differential diagnostic clue is the complete absence of vessels and enhancement in the central liquid portion of an abscess, while even hypovascular metastases will display some weak but visible central enhancement due to small vessels, provided they are not necrotic.

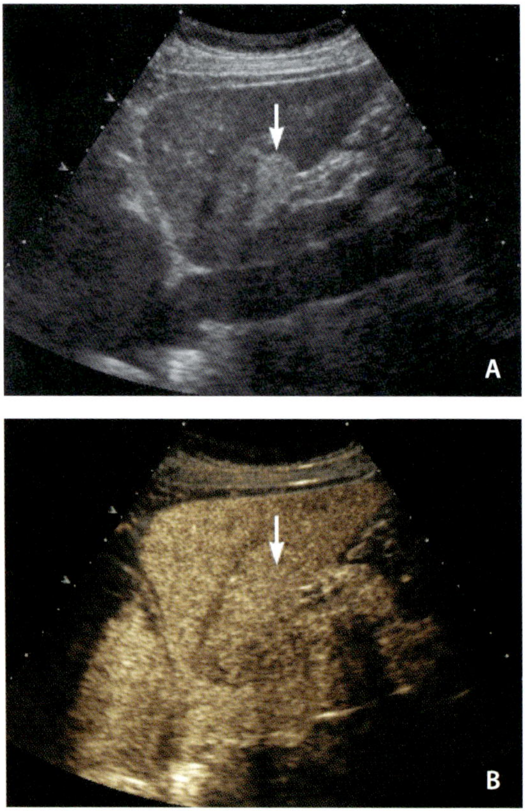

Fig. 12. Focal fatty infiltration (*arrow*) in a patient on chemotherapy for breast cancer. **A** B-mode US shows a triangular hyperechoic lesion in segment III. **B** Delayed-phase imaging after SonoVue administration shows normal enhancement of the lesion which has disappeared. Note: with this imaging technique (Cadence Contrast Pulse Sequencing, CPS, Siemens, Mountain View, CA, USA), one identical US frame can be displayed either as a "tissue only" image without contrast information (**A**) or as a "mixed" image with the contrast information superimposed, which is displayed in colour (**B**)

Clinical Results

In a recently published study [8], we addressed the question of whether the characterisation of focal liver lesions can be improved by dynamic SonoVue-enhanced low-MI real-time contrast-specific US in comparison to baseline US (including unenhanced grey-scale and power Doppler US).

Sixty-three patients were included and one lesion per patient was evaluated. The final lesion diagnosis was based on histology findings in 25 cases and on unequivocal imaging findings on MRI (n=19), CT (n=18) or intraoperative US (n=1) in the remaining 38 patients. In 11 patients with lesion characterisation based on imaging, confirmatory follow-up imaging data were available. The lesions studied were 27 metastases, 6 HCCs, 2 cholangiocarcinomas, 11 haemangiomas, 11 FNHs, 3 areas of focal fatty change/sparing, 2 regenerating nodules and 1 abscess.

Ten of the 27 metastases were "hypervascular" on arterial phase imaging with homogeneous enhancement; the primaries in these patients were malignant melanoma (n=6), small cell lung cancer, thyroid carcinoma, neuroendocrine carcinoma and breast cancer (one each). The remaining 18 metastases were "hypovascular" and showed either a rim enhancement (n=10) or no enhancement at all (n=7) in the arterial phase; the most common primaries in this group were colorectal (n=9) and bronchogenic carcinoma (n=3). In the portal venous and delayed phase all 27 metastases were hypoechoic compared to normal liver. On baseline US, 25 (93%) metastases were correctly diagnosed; after contrast administration, all 27 (100%) metastases were recognised.

Six CCCs were studied and there was intense arterial enhancement in all these lesions. During the portal venous and delayed liver phase, three of the lesions were mostly hyporeflective and two slightly hyporeflective (Fig. 2), while the remaining one HCC was isoreflective.

Two CCCs were included: in the arterial phase one of these showed rim enhancement and there was no arterial enhancement in the other. In the portal venous and delayed phase both lesions produced hyporeflective enhancement defects.

In summary, 34 (97 %) of the 35 reference-proven malignant lesions appeared hyporeflective in the portal venous and delayed phase. Twenty-eight of the lesions were benign; correct diagnosis of benignity was made in 12 (43%) of these on baseline and in 25 (89%) after contrast enhancement. Two benign lesions were misinterpreted as malignant after contrast enhancement: one abscess and one atypical haemangioma which did not fill with contrast agent after the arterial phase. One regenerating nodule remained unclear.

In conclusion, the study showed marked improvement in characterisation of focal liver lesions by the use of SonoVue. Overall, the number of correctly diagnosed lesions improved from 41 of 63 (65%) on baseline US to 58 (92%) after contrast agent administration ($p<0.001$). Comparison with the literature suggests that CEUS is superior to CT and probably equivalent to MRI in this application [9-11]. The most important aspect of these results with regards to imaging cancer patients is the increase in specificity, i.e. the improved ability to recognise benign lesions and to rule out metastases.

Limitations

The same limitations that apply to conventional US also apply to CEUS. Any patient that has difficult sonographic access to the liver because of obesity or otherwise unfavourable anatomy will also be difficult to image with contrast agents. Particularly problematic are patients with severe steatosis and limited penetration of sound into the liver. In such cases it is often not possible to see contrast enhancement beyond a few centimetres in depth, which is usually not sufficient for diagnosis.

Conclusion

Until recently, US was the preferred screening method for focal liver lesions disease because of its inherent advantages; however, it suffered from relatively poor sensitivity and specificity compared with other imaging techniques such as CT and MRI and further imaging was often required for a definitive diagnosis if a lesion was seen on conventional US.

Since the advent of US contrast agents and new contrast-specific US techniques, liver US has dramatically evolved. Lesion characterisation is markedly improved. The ability of contrast US to characterise focal liver lesions is superior to that of CT and similar to that of MRI. CEUS is now the imaging modality of choice for characterisation of any focal liver lesions since it is quick, inexpensive, well tolerated by patients and highly accurate. On the other hand, some limitations of US remain, such as its operator dependence and the limited access to certain parts of the liver especially in obese patients and/or fatty livers.

CEUS is a young field that continues to progress rapidly. It adds a new dimension to liver US and has become a pivotal part of liver imaging in our daily practice as it provides us with crucial diagnostic information that is completely occult to conventional sonography. CEUS of the liver can be used as an alternative or, in difficult cases, as an adjunct to CT and MRI.

References

1. Edmunson H, Craig J (1987) Neoplasms of the liver. In: Schiff L (ed) Diseases of the liver, 8th edn. Lippincott, Philadelphia pp 1109
2. Cosgrove DO (2001) Malignant Liver disease. In: Meire HB, Cosgrove DO, Dewbury KC, Farrant P (eds) Clinical ultrasound a comprehensive text. Abdominal and general ultrasound, 2nd edn. Churchill Livingstone, London vol 1:211-231
3. Karhunen PJ (1986) Benign hepatic tumours and tumour like conditions in men. J Clin Pathol 39:183-188
4. Jones EC, Chezmar JL, Nelson RC, Bernardino ME (1992) The frequency and significance of small (less than or equal to 15 mm) hepatic lesions detected by CT. AJR Am J Roentgenol 158:535-539
5. Kreft B, Pauleit D, Bachmann R et al (2001) Häufigkeit und Bedeutung von kleinen fokalen Leberläsionen. Rofo Fortschr Geb Rontgenstr Neuen Bildgeb Verfahr 173:424-429
6. Ishak KG, Rabin L (1975) Benign tumors of the liver. Med Clin North Am 59:995-1013
7. Wanless IR, Albrecht S, Bilbao J et al (1989) Multiple focal nodular hyperplasia of the liver associated with vascular malformations of various organs and neoplasia of the brain: a new syndrome. Mod Pathol 2:456-462
8. Hohmann J, Skrok J, Puls R, Albrecht T (2003) Characterization of focal liver lesions with contrast-enhanced low MI real time ultrasound and SonoVue. Rofo Fortschr Geb Rontgenstr Neuen Bildgeb Verfahr 175:835-843
9. Oudkerk M, van Beek EJ, Wielopolski P et al (2002) Comparison of contrast-enhanced magnetic resonance angiography and conventional pulmonary angiography for the diagnosis of pulmonary embolism: a prospective study. Lancet 359:1643-1647
10. Pirovano G, Vanzulli A, Marti-Bonmati L et al (2000) Evaluation of the accuracy of gadobenate dimeglumine-enhanced MR imaging in the detection and characterization of focal liver lesions. AJR Am J Roentgenol 175:1111-1120
11. Semelka RC, Martin DR, Balci C, Lance T (2001) Focal liver lesions: comparison of dual-phase CT and multisequence multiplanar MR imaging including dynamic gadolinium enhancement. J Magn Reson Imaging 13:397-401

Lars Thorelius

Chapter 2

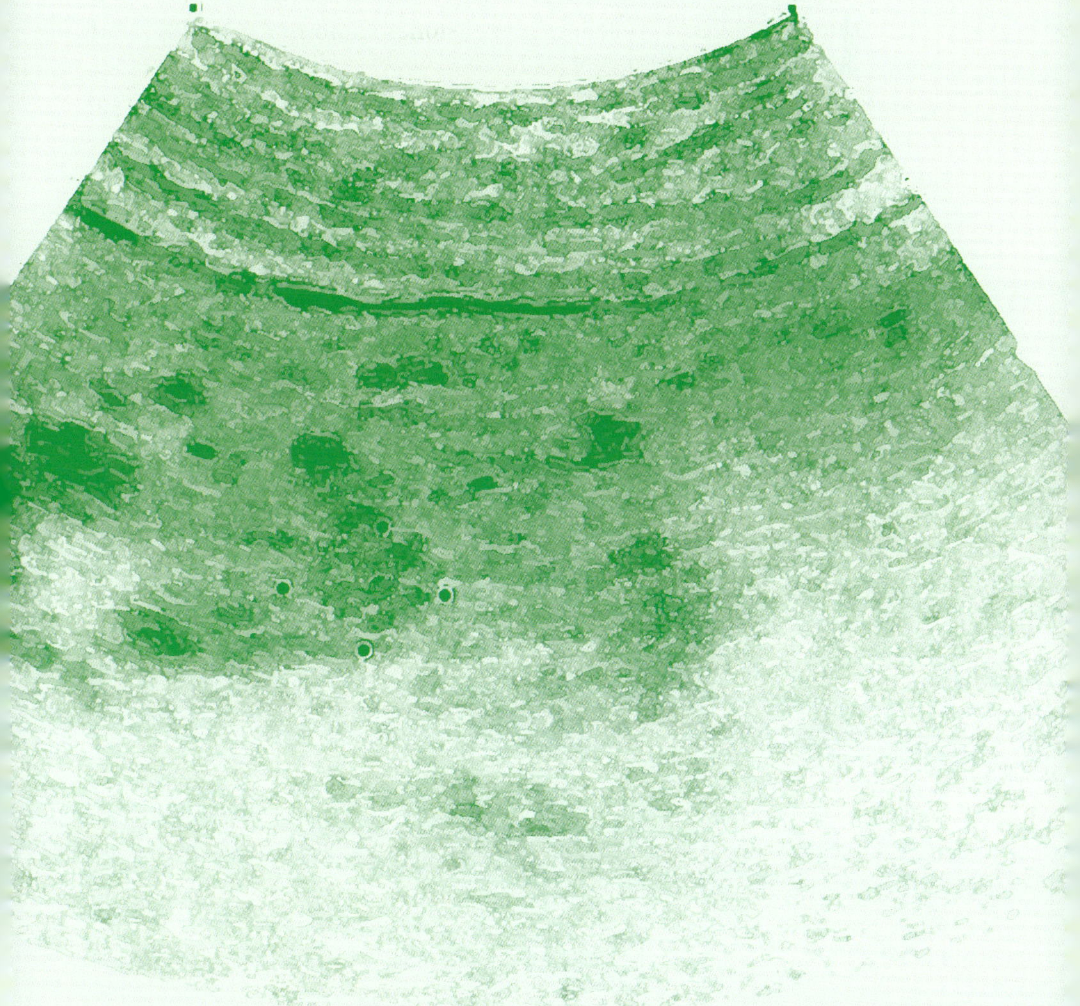

Usefulness of Contrast-Enhanced Ultrasound in the Characterization of Pancreatic and Renal Masses

Lars Thorelius
Department of Radiology, University Hospital Linköping,
Linköping, Sweden

A case series of pancreatic and renal masses is presented to illustrate the usefulness of contrast-enhanced ultrasound with SonoVue in the visualization of these lesions. The technique appears to depict pancreatic vascularity particularly well, providing useful diagnostic information for vascular diagnoses, as well as additional information on the extent of viable tissue and the ideal site for a biopsy. It is also a promising technique for the detection of small, necrotic lesions, infarction and traumatic hematomas in the kidney.

Several articles in the literature have convincingly reported on the usefulness of echocontrast agents for the detection and characterization of focal liver lesions [1-6]. In our center, based on the experience gained using contrast agents for liver imaging, we are now trying to acquire a better knowledge of the behavior and possible utilization of contrast also for non-liver applications. The following is a summary of our experience in visualizing pancreatic and renal masses with contrast-enhanced ultrasound (CEUS) with a second-generation contrast agent, SonoVue (Bracco Imaging, Italy), as compared to other imaging modalities.

Materials

In almost all cases of non-liver imaging, we use Acuson Sequoia ultrasound machines equipped with CPS (Siemens, USA), which is a special software that is designed to detect the non-linear fundamental response of microbubbles. One advantage of this system is the possibility to separate the gray-scale image from the contrast image; this facilitates the distinction between vascular and non-vascular areas. We have found that 1.2 ml of SonoVue is often the correct bolus volume for imaging of abdominal structures other than the liver and spleen. However, the kidneys enhance very intensely, and the standard bolus for the adult kidney is no more than 0.6 ml.

Pancreatic Masses

In the pancreas, uptake of contrast medium during CEUS using SonoVue is very rapid; at approximately 25-40 s it produces a transient, bright homogeneous enhancement that is due to the high vascularization of the organ. Accumulation in the capillaries is negligible, thus the washout also occurs rapidly after the arterial phase, giving the pancreas a darkened appearance in contrast to the adjacent liver after 2 min. Consequently, CEUS is not very good at delineating masses, but it does permit good delineation of non-vascular pancreatic lesions.

Non-enhanced ultrasound (US) is underestimated for the delineation of pancreatic masses. An example of a well-delineated necrotic tumor is shown in Fig. 1.

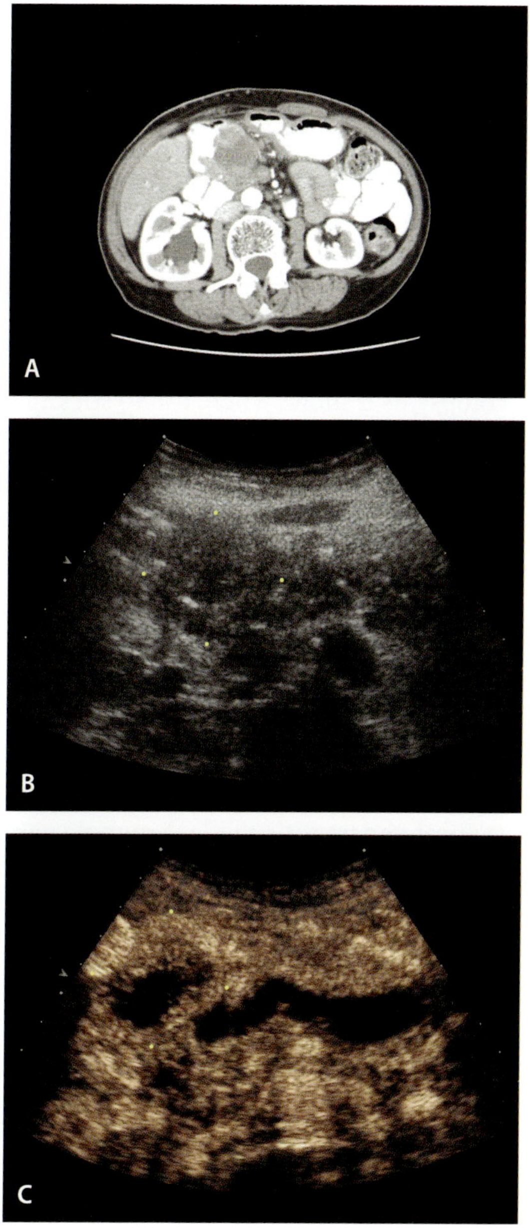

Fig. 1. A CT of pancreas cancer. **B** US of pancreatic cancer (marked by yellow dots). **C** CEUS of pancreas cancer (marked by yellow dots)

CT depicts the tumor covering the entire head of the pancreas, which is also well delineated as a rounded mass on non-enhanced US images (small tumors can actually often be visualized better by non-enhanced US than CT).

When the image of the large mass was enhanced by injecting SonoVue, the necrotic area became much smaller, showing that the vascularization of the tumor was more widespread than what appeared on the CT images. The key information provided by CEUS was therefore not the delineation of the mass, but the delineation of viable tissue and vascularization, which is valuable information for the performance of a biopsy, as it shows where not to stick the needle.

After injection of contrast, small tumors are actually drowned by contrast material, so in this case CEUS is not helpful.

On the other hand, CEUS can be useful in focal pancreatitis, in which non-vascular necrotic tissue can easily be visualized in contrast to vascular surrounding tissue. In a case of acute abdominal pain, CEUS was useful in revealing a non-enhancing wedge-shaped area that looked like a small focal pancreatitis, but was an area of necrotic pancreatitis. However, when the area of pancreatitis is large, no additional information is provided by CEUS, as shown in Fig. 2: the injection of contrast in a patient who suffered an episode of acute, severe focal pancreatitis made the whole pancreas echoic, thus not adding more information than non-enhanced US.

In our experience, CEUS is so far also not useful in rare tumors of the pancreas, such as insulinoma. In the case presented in Fig. 3, a 15-mm-wide mass corresponding to an insulinoma was beautifully delineated by non-enhanced US. Contrast material really drowned the mass, making it less visible. CT also did not provide clear images of this mass, so the best modality in this case was non-enhanced US.

One case is one of von Hippel-Lindau's disease, which is a rare genetic entity characterized by angiomatosis and hemangioblastomas. In one of our cases (Fig. 4) there was concern that a small dot was an aneurysm rather than a capillary tumor. CT did not permit the visualization of the entrance of contrast medium with reference to other tissues, whereas CEUS did. After the injection of SonoVue, the arteries filled first and permitted detailed visualization of pancreatic vascularity with excellent temporal resolution, which enabled us to conclude that the diagnosis was most likely a capillary tumor rather than an aneurysm.

Thus, when it comes to the pancreas, CEUS does not provide much information about the actual masses, but the detailed visualization of vascularity can be very useful to establish the extent of viable tissue, where to perform a biopsy and to formulate vascular diagnoses.

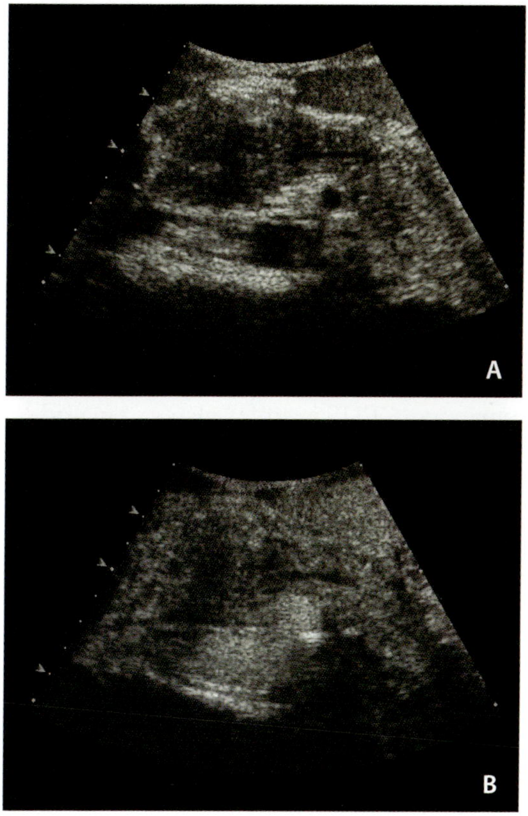

Fig. 2. A US of acute focal pancreatitis. **B** CEUS of acute focal pancreatitis

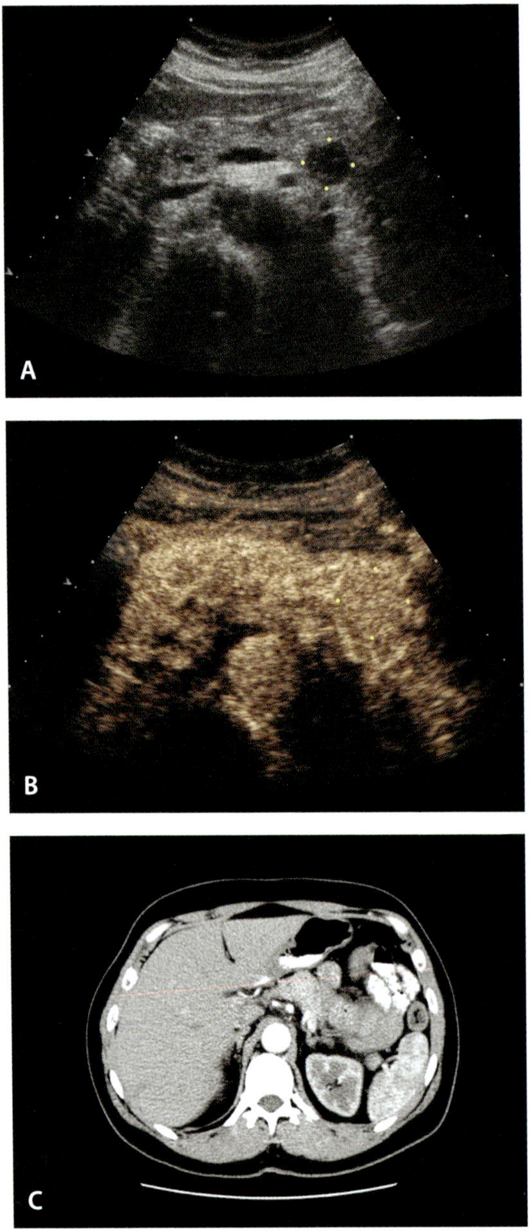

Fig. 3. A US of insulinoma. **B** CEUS of insulinoma. **C** CT of insulinoma

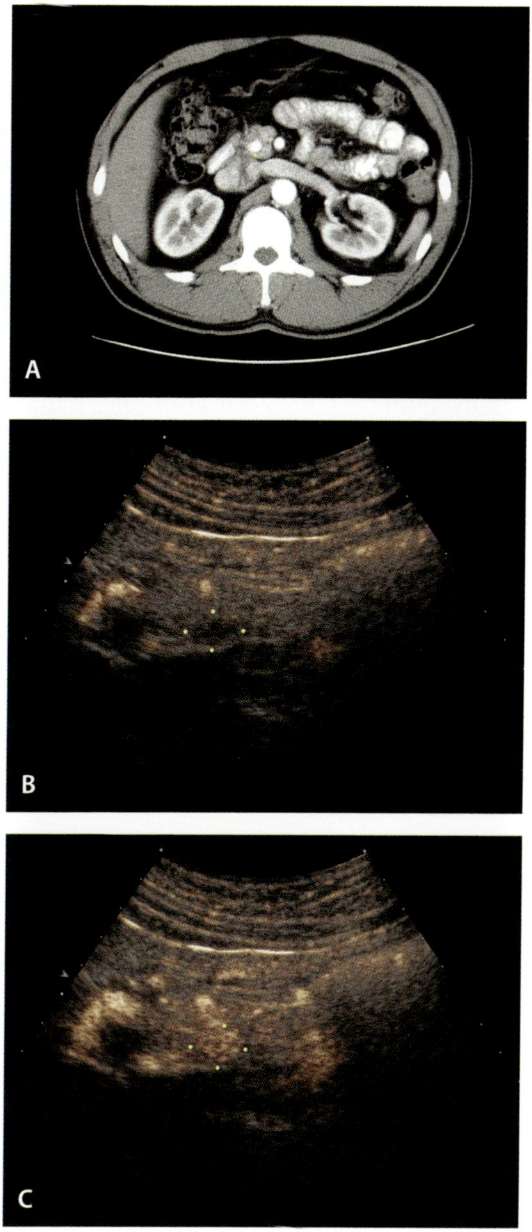

Fig. 4. A CT of capillary tumor (yellow dot). **B** CEUS of capillary tumor after artery enhancement but not yet of tumor. **C** CEUS 3 s later, with enhancement of capillary tumor

Renal Masses

CEUS of the kidney provides a clear and detailed view of renal vascularity, with early enhancement in the arterial phase followed by an intense and uniform enhancement in the renal cortex. Enhancement then extends to the pyramids until they become isoechoic with the cortex, about 20-30 s later.

The enhancement, which lasts about 2 minutes and then gradually fades, is produced by concentration of contrast medium in the arteries; accumulation of contrast medium in the parenchyma is negligible. Consequently, CEUS does not offer a major advantage over non-enhanced US in the detection and characterization of focal renal lesions. Moreover, contrast medium does not concentrate in the urine as it does in urograms and CT examinations.

In most cases, CEUS does not provide more details about renal tumors than non-enhanced US. However, it can reveal necrotic areas and can therefore be very useful in the detection of small, necrotic tumors, which are difficult to see with non-enhanced US.

Angiomyolipomas are surprisingly vascularized; after injection of contrast material, even angiolipomas may be difficult to distinguish from the rest of the kidney in any of the phases.

Hematomas, on the other hand, are readily distinguished from other tissues. A case of postoperative pain after lithotripsy is presented in Fig. 5. The urogram detected an unexplained mass and CEUS revealed a non-enhancing subcapsular mass that could be identified as a hematoma.

We draw the conclusion that when there is no enhancement during CEUS, there is no risk of finding a viable tumor in the area.

Small infarctions can also be difficult to assess with other modalities. In Fig. 6 the case of a patient with flank pain is presented, in whom contrast-enhanced CT showed a probable infarction, but it was not clear. CEUS revealed an area devoid of contrast with sharp margins that could easily be identified as a renal infarction.

In our region of Sweden there are quite a few cases of hereditary renal cancers. Both patients and relatives undergo imaging investigations to rule out the development of aggressive papillary tumors. We subjected them to CEUS to see whether this novel imaging modality would provide more information.

The tumors were surprisingly poorly vascularized and appeared as small hypoechoic dots. Thus, CEUS was able to detect very small lesions – potential applications of this ability will be pursued and investigated further.

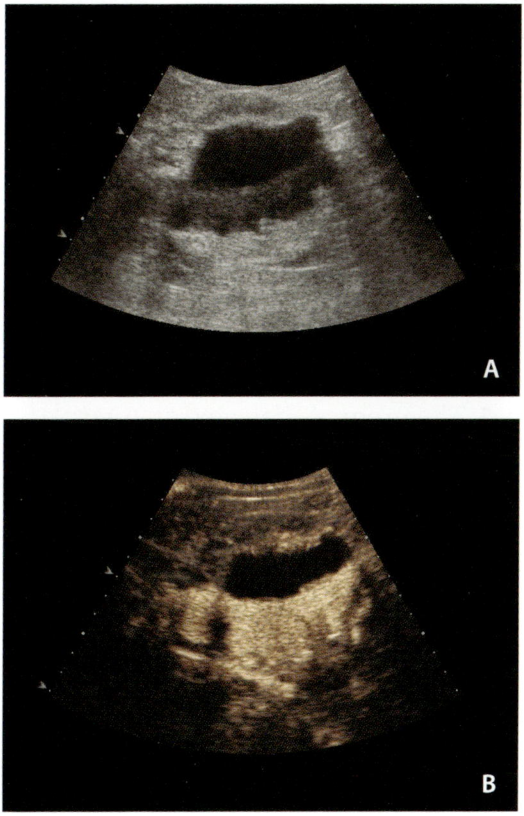

Fig. 5. A US of renal hematoma. **B** CEUS of renal hematoma

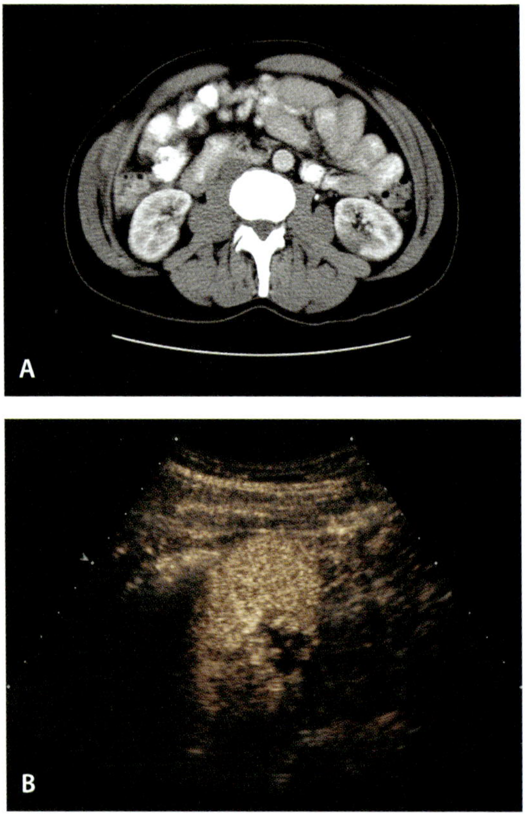

Fig. 6. A CT of probable infarction in left kidney. **B** CEUS of obvious infarction

Conclusion

In summary, CEUS is a promising technique for the detection of small, necrotic lesions, infarction and hematomas due to trauma of the kidney [7]. It does not appear to have efficient potential in the visualization of small, highly vascular renal tumors, such as small hypernephromas; however, one promising area is that of surveillance of hereditary cancers with low vascularization.

References

1. Quaia E, Callida F, Bertolotto M et al (2004) Characterization of Focal Liver Lesions with Contrast-specific US Modes and a Sulfur Hexafluoride-filled Microbubble Contrast Agent: Diagnostic Performance and Confidence. Radiology 232(2):420-430
2. Hohmann J, Skrok J, Puls R, Albrecht T (2004) Characterization of Focal Liver Lesions with Contrast-enhanced Low MI Real Time Ultrasound and SonoVue. Fortschr Röntgenstr 176:1-9
3. Hohmann J, Albrecht T, Oldenburg A et al (2004) Liver metastases in cancer: detection with contrast-enhanced ultrasonography. Abdom Imaging 29/6:669-681
4. Gaiani S, Celli N, Piscaglia F et al (2004) Usefulness of contrast-enhanced perfusional sonography in the assessment of hepatocellular carcinoma hypervascular at spiral computed tomography. J Hepatol 4(3):421-426
5. Quaia E, Stacul F, Gaiani S et al (2004) Comparison of diagnostic performance of unenhanced vs SonoVue - enhanced ultrasonography in focal liver lesions characterization. The experience of three Italian centers. Radiol Med 108(1-2):71-81
6. Dietrich CF (2004) Characterisation of focal liver lesions with contrast enhanced ultrasonography. Eur J Radiol 51(Suppl):S9-17
7. Thorelius L (2004) Contrast-enhanced ultrasound for extrahepatic lesions: preliminary experience. Eur J Radiol 51(Suppl):S31-38

Luigi Solbiati, Luca Cova

Chapter 3

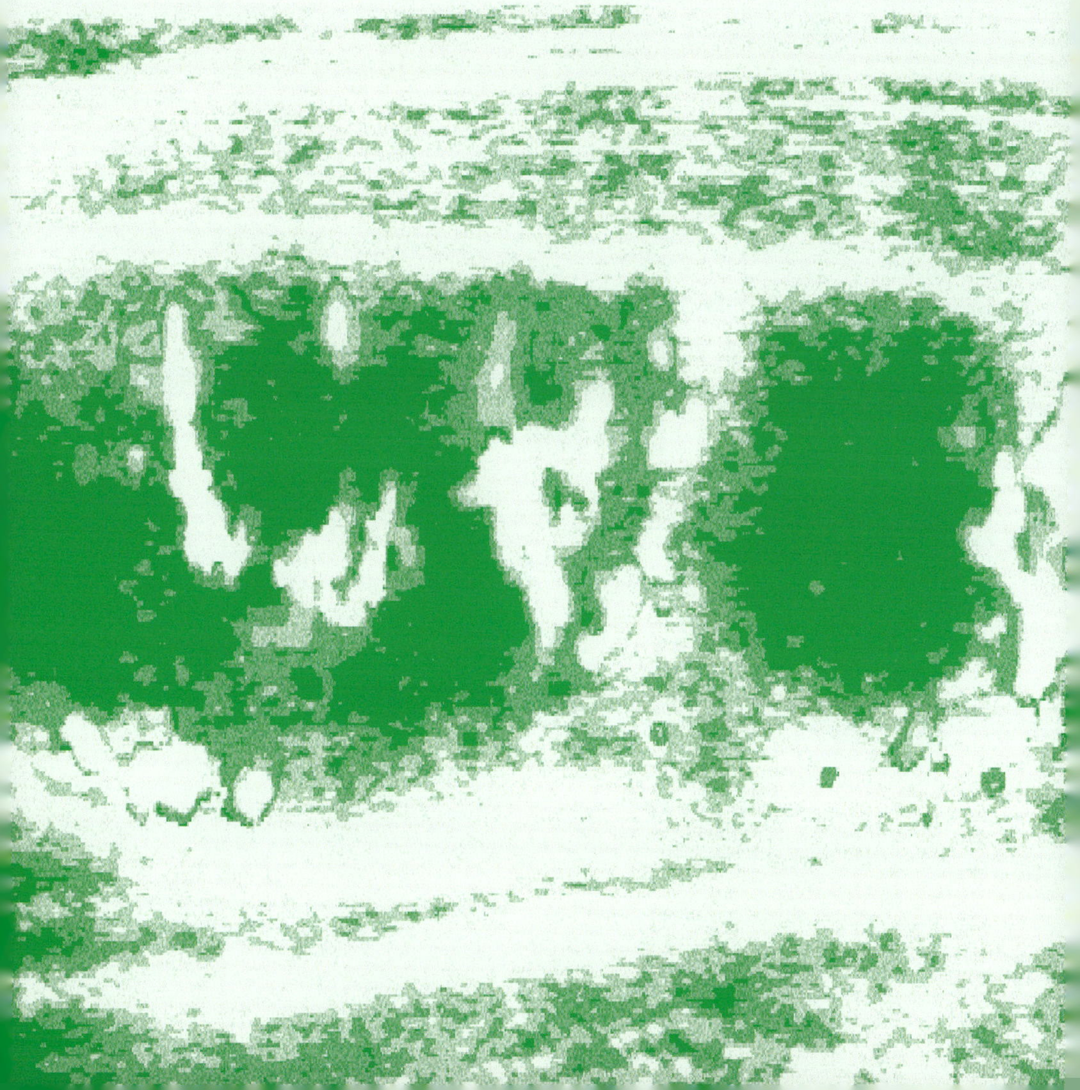

Improved Characterization of Reactive and Malignant Lymph Nodes Using Contrast-Enhanced Ultrasound

LUIGI SOLBIATI, LUCA COVA
Department of Radiology, General Hospital
Busto Arsizio, Varese, Italy

Introduction

Contrast-enhanced ultrasound (CEUS), using second generation contrast agents such as SonoVue, permits the use of the low mechanical index required for the detailed visualization of the vascularity of lymph nodes which can be detected with gray-scale harmonic imaging techniques. These techniques allow real-time analysis of all vascular phases and the visualization of intranodal focal "avascular" areas that represent deposits of neoplastic cells or necrosis. Preliminary data suggest that this novel imaging modality can improve the differential diagnosis of malignant lymph nodes from reactive nodes and provide a more accurate selection of nodes to be submitted to fine-needle aspiration biopsy. In addition, the simultaneous assessment of macro- and micro-vascularity may enable the detection of new diagnostic features that cannot be visualized with other imaging modalities, such as "spotty" enhancement of lymphomas. Further studies are needed to validate these features.

For many years, lymph nodes have been assessed with traditional ultrasound (US) technology using morphological criteria, such as size (thickness), shape (the ratio between the longitudinal and short-axis), hyperechoic hilus, echogenicity of the cortex, calcifications and intranodal necrotic or cystic changes [1-8].

Subsequently, vascularity criteria were added, differentiating between nodes with a visible hilus, focal absence of perfusion, and the presence of subcapsular, displaced and/or burnt vessels (Tschammler's classification) [9] by means of color and power Doppler. This improved the ability to differentiate neoplastic from reactive nodes, yielding a diagnostic sensitivity of 83-89% and a specificity of 87-93% (87-98%) [8]. However, although normal or reactive nodes usually have hilar vascularity, in as many as 35% of cases they do not show any vascularity, especially when the short axis is under 3-4 mm. In addition, with color and power Doppler, further problems may occur: lack of flow signals in deeply located nodes, artifacts in nodes adjacent to large vessels, failure to visualize microvascularity and, more importantly, no depiction of focal avascular changes representing necrosis or metastatic deposits [8-14].

Contrast-enhanced ultrasound (CEUS) for the investigation of lymph nodes has recently become available. Very few papers have been published on its use so far [15-18].

CEUS using color Doppler and first-generation contrast agents was superior to computed tomography (CT) and magnetic resonance imaging (MRI) in terms of diagnostic accuracy [15]. In a study on 94 enlarged lymph nodes in 39 adults with carcinoma of the oral cavity, the vascularity was depicted in 86% of the nodes; in 28%, unenhanced B-mode US was unable to depict the vessels. The diagnosis changed in 14% of cases and led to changes in therapy in 4% [16].

However, first-generation contrast agents are not suitable for-low mechanical index (MI) settings, which are necessary for the visualization of the slow flow in small structures, such as lymph nodes. Currently, second-generation contrast agents permit the use of low

MI and can be detected with gray-scale harmonic imaging techniques, thus allowing real-time analysis of all vascular phases, including the parenchymal phase; therefore, they provide extremely detailed information on the perfusion of lymph nodes [17].

We used two different systems enabling the study of superficial nodes with high frequency and microbubbles: one based on harmonics (CnTi, Esaote) and one based on the changes in fundamental frequency amplitude signals (CPS, Acuson Siemens), both used with low MI (0.05-0.2) in continuous mode.

We administered a second-generation contrast medium, SonoVue (Bracco Imaging SpA, Milan, Italy), made of microbubbles containing sulfur hexafluoride stabilized by a highly elastic phospholipids monolayer, with outstanding stability and resistance to US pressure [19]. A single intravenous dose was given (2.4-4.8 ml); the total vial (4.8 ml) was usually necessary to study large, deeply located nodes.

Different patterns of enhancement (both for morphology and timing of enhancement) were observed for the different histologic types of adenopathy.

Normal and reactive lymph nodes (Fig.1)

Anatomically, the blood supply of normal/reactive nodes enters via the hilar artery to the small arteries of the medulla, ending in the sinuous capillaries of the nodal cortex. Whereas color and power Doppler US can usually depict the hilar vascularity, but not the whole arterial system [1, 11], enhancement of the hilus is seen on CEUS at 10-15 s following bolus injection, followed at 15-25 s by homogeneous enhancement of either macro- and microvascularity of the cortex. Wash-out starts at 40-45 s and is usually complete after 60-90 s.

When reactive nodes have extensive fatty changes, the hilus is enhanced, whereas the cortex remains homogeneously avascular.

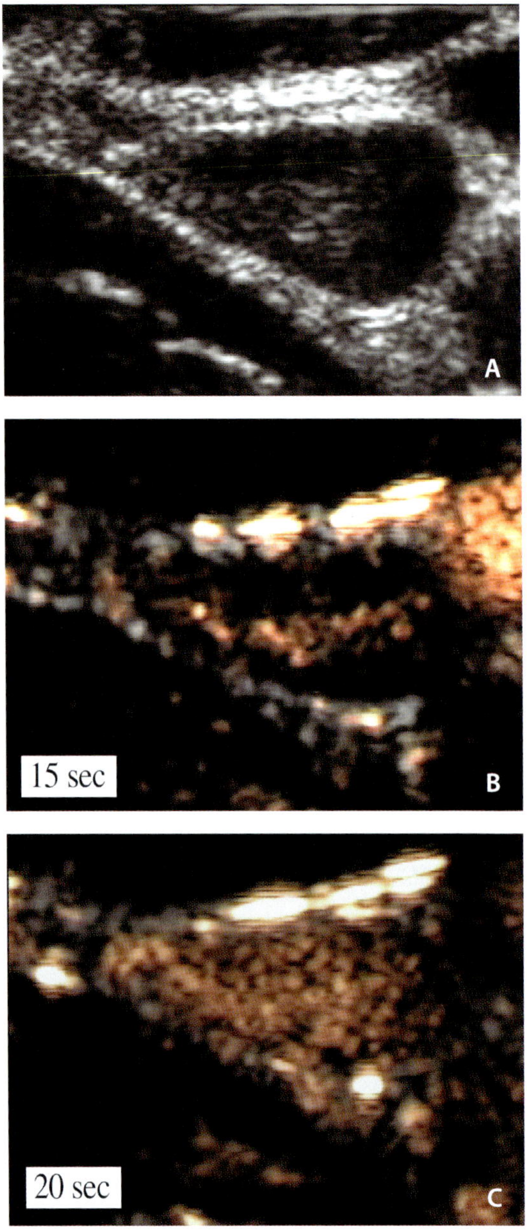

Fig. 1. 7-mm reactive node of the laterocervical chain on B-mode sonography (**A**). On CEUS, at 15 s after bolus injection of SonoVue, only the centrally located hilus is enhanced (**B**). At 20 s completely homogeneous enhancement of the nodal cortex is seen (**C**)

Granulomatous adenitis (Fig. 2)

In the few cases of granulomatous adenitis we have examined to date with CEUS using SonoVue, the hilus is thin and quickly enhancing and the cortex is homogeneously vascularized, but with a "grainy" pattern which seems to be a characteristic feature of granulomatous nodes (Fig. 2).

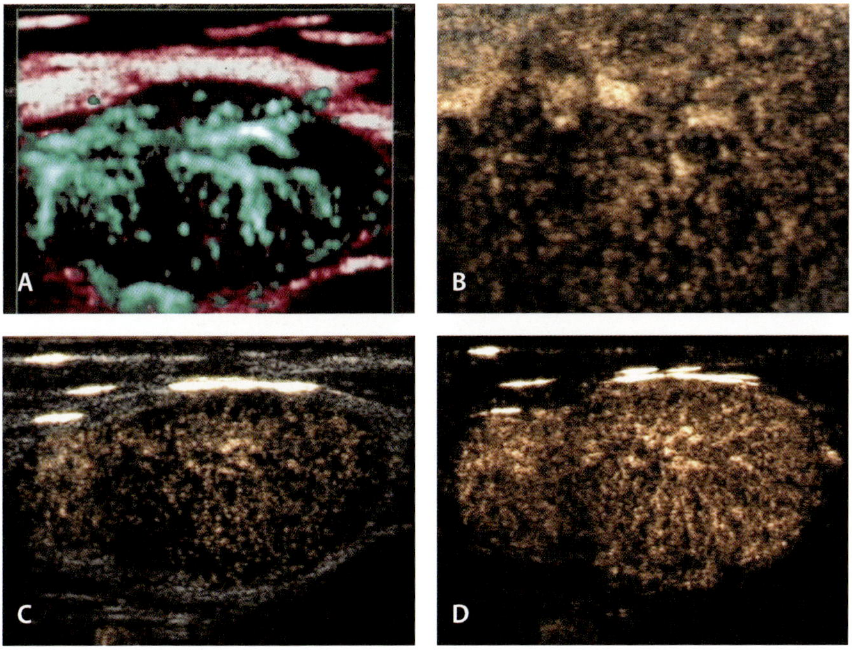

Fig. 2. Granulomatous adenitis. After bolus injection of SonoVue, at 15 s only the hilar vascularity is seen with regular arrangement (**A**). At 20 s (**B**), 25 s (**C**) and 40 s (**D**) progressive enhancement of the nodal cortex is seen with a likely characteristic "grainy" pattern

Metastatic nodes (Figs. 3, 4)

Pathologically, in metastatic nodes infiltration by tumoral cells distorts and destroys nodal vascular structure, including hilar blood vessels. In addition, neoplastic infiltration of the cortex associated with angiogenesis and recruitment of capsular vessels leads to peripheral hypervascularity with tortuous and aberrant feeding vessels at the periphery and sinusoid neovascularity within the tumoral nests. Thus, central perfusion predominates in benign nodes and peripheral perfusion in malignant nodes. This difference can often be detected with color and power Doppler, but sinusoid neovascularity within the tumor nests cannot be depicted [10-12].

With CEUS using SonoVue, enhancement of capsular vessels is seen at 10-15 s, followed by the appearance of internal aberrant and usually tortuous blood vessels, whereas the hilus is undetectable. At 15-25 s, inhomogeneous enhancement of the cortex appears, with focal hypoechoic changes due to hypovascular or avascular (necrotic changes) metastatic deposits. At 40-60 s washout starts and hypoechoic foci are no longer visible.

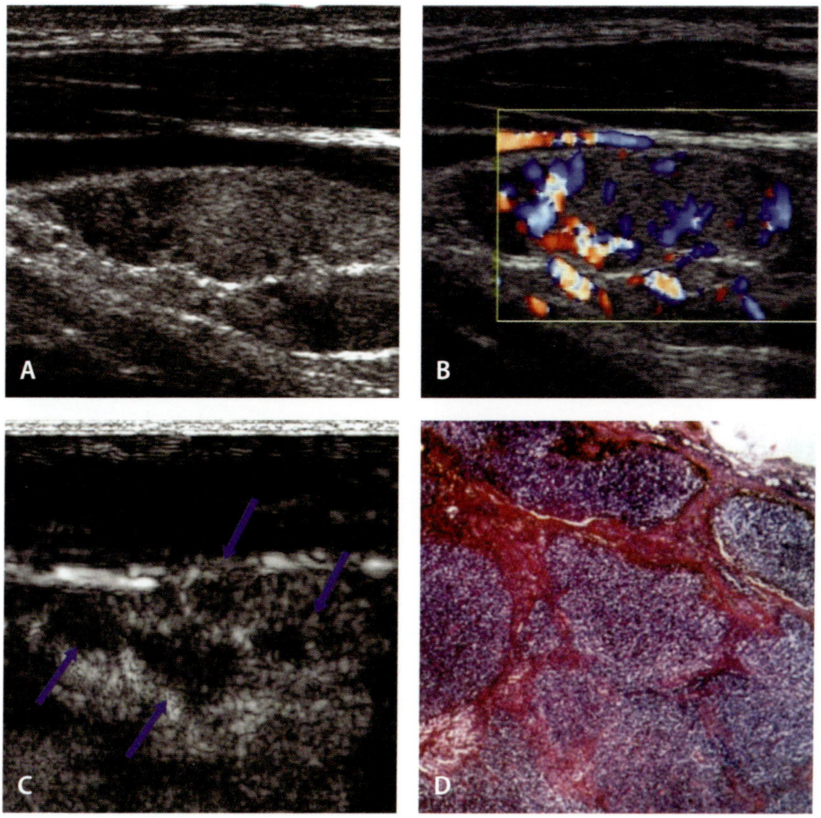

Fig. 3. Example of large, oval, hyperechoic metastatic node (**A**). Color Doppler shows flow signals in the cranial portion of the adenopathy, while the caudal portion seems completely avascular (**B**). On the contrary, in the parenchymal phase after injection of SonoVue, many hypovascular areas (**C**) corresponding to the metastatic deposits detectable in the histological specimen (**D**) are seen

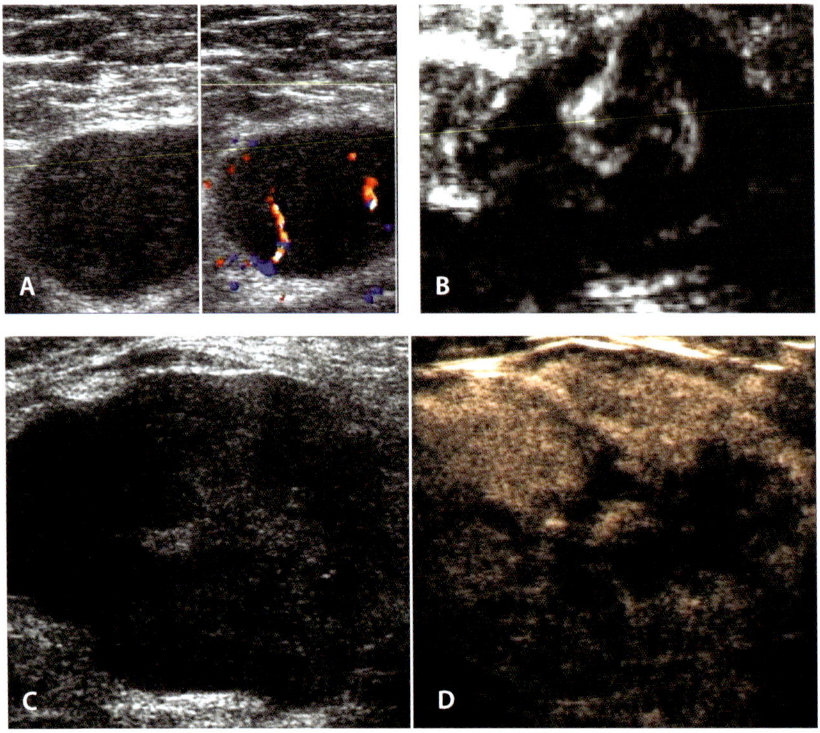

Fig. 4. Two adjacent metastatic nodes. In the first node (**A**, left) only a few scattered flow signals are seen on color Doppler (**A**, right), whereas CEUS (**B**) demonstrates tortuous blood vessels and hypovascular areas at the peripehry. In the second node (**C**), CEUS shows a very large internal necrotic area and irregular margins which are features of malignant nature (**D**)

Lymphomatous nodes (Fig. 5)

As demonstrated in previous reports [17, 18] in the few cases of lymphomatous nodes studied in our series, in arterial phase (10-15 s.) macrovascularity is poorly visualized and the hilus is very thin, usually undetectable and displaced to the periphery of the node. Parenchymal enhancement starts with diffuse bright spots ("snow-like" appearance), which subsequently fuse, leading to homogenous enhancement. This pattern has not been observed in any other nodal disease with CEUS.

In Hodgkin's lymphomas of nodular sclerosis type, extremely rounded and very well demarcated avascular or hypovascular intraparenchymal areas are frequently seen, as shown in Figure 5.

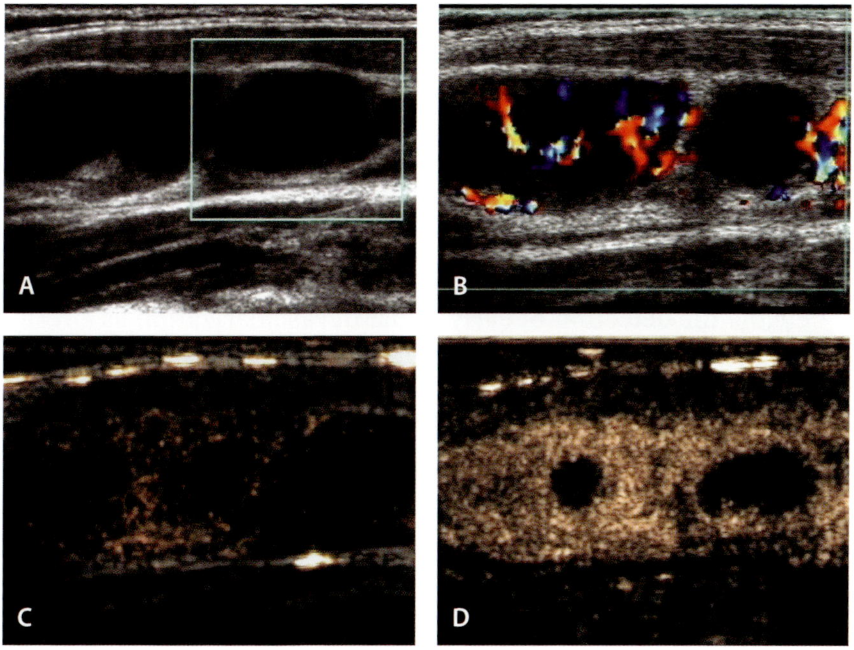

Fig. 5. Two adjacent nodes affected with Hodgkin's lymphoma of nodular sclerosis type. Marked hypoechogenicity is shown on B-mode sonography (**A**) and very few blood flow signals are depicted with color Doppler (**B**). With CEUS, very slow enhancement is seen in arterial phase (**C**), while in venous phase (**D**) the parenchymal enhancement is inhomogeneous due to the presence of multiple rounded avascular foci

Conclusions

Real-time study of all vascular phases, visualization of microvascularity in each lymph node independently of its size, and detection of intranodal focal "avascular" areas representing deposits of neoplastic cells or necrotic changes are the three most important advancements achievable with CEUS and second-generation contrast agents.

The simultaneous assessment of macro- and micro-vascularity may enable the detection of "new" diagnostic features, such as "spotty" enhancement of lymphomas and focal avascular areas in metastatic modes which need to be validated in further studies.

Fine-needle aspiration biopsy (FNAB) remains the main diagnostic modality for lymph nodes. However, currently adopted diagnostic criteria for US, CT, and MRI show limitations in the detection of small non-necrotic metastases in normal-sized or slightly enlarged nodes, and multiple FNABs may be necessary [12, 20]. The study of the microvascularity of even normal-sized nodes with CEUS may enable more accurate selection of nodes to be submitted to FNAB, thereby reducing the number of pathologic assessments.

The assessment of nodal microvascular enhancement may also enable the detection of early nodal devascularization as a result of chemo- and/or radiation therapy. Consequently, CEUS might be used to achieve early, easy, and confident assessment of the therapeutic response of both lymphomatous and squamous-cell carcinomas to radiation treatment and/or chemotherapy.

References

1. Vassallo P, Wernecke K, Roos N, Peters PE (1992) Differentiation of benign from malignant superficial lymphadenopathy: the role of high-resolution US. Radiology 183:215-220
2. Solbiati L, Cioffi V, Ballarati E (1992) Ultrasonography of the neck. Radiol Clin North Am 30:941-954
3. Bruneton JN, Maestro C, Marcy PY, Padovani B (1994) Echography of the superficial lymph nodes. J Radiol 75: 373-381
4. Ying M, Ahuja A, Brook F et al (1996) Sonographic appearance and distribution of normal cervical lymph nodes in a Chinese population. J Ultrasound Med 15:431-436
5. Mancuso AA, Harnsberger HR, Muraki AS, Stevens MH (1983) Computed tomography of cervical and retropharyngeal lymph nodes: normal anatomy, variants of normal, and applications in staging head and neck cancer. Part I: normal anatomy. Radiology 148:709-714
6. Mancuso AA, Harnsberger HR, Muraki AS, Stevens MH (1983) Computed tomography of cervical and retropharyngeal lymph nodes: normal anatomy, variants of normal, and applications in staging head and neck cancer. Part II: pathology. Radiology 148:715-723
7. Som PM (1987) Lymph nodes of the neck. Radiology 165:593-600
8. Ahuja A, Ying M (2003) Sonography of neck lymph nodes. Part II: abnormal lymph nodes. Clin Radiol 58:359-366
9. Tschammler A, Ott G, Schang T et al (1998) Lymphadenopathy: differentiation of benign from malignant disease. Color Doppler US assessment of intranodal angioarchitecture. Radiology 208:117-123
10. Wu CH, Shih JC, Chang YL et al (1998) Two-dimensional and three-dimensional power Doppler sonographic classification of vascular patterns in cervical lymphadenopathies. J Ultrasound Med 17:459-464
11. Na DG, Lim HK, Byun HS et al (1997) Differential diagnosis of cervical lymphadenopathy: usefulness of color Doppler Sonography. AJR 168:1311-1316
12. Steinkamp HJ, Wissgott C, Rademaker J, Felix R (2002) Current status of power Doppler and color Doppler sonography in the differential diagnosis of lymph node lesions. Eur Radiol 12:1785-1793
13. Ariji Y, Kimura Y, Hayashi N et al (1998) Power Doppler Sonography of cervical lymph nodes in patients with head and neck cancer. Am J Neuroradiol 19:303-307

14. Wu CH, Chang YL, Hsu WC et al (1998) Usefulness of Doppler spectral analysis and power Doppler sonography in the differentiation of cervical lymphadenopathies. AJR 171:503-509
15. Moritz JD, Ludwig A, Oestmann JW (2000) Contrast-enhanced color Doppler sonography for evaluation of enlarged cervical lymph nodes in head and neck tumors. AJR 174:1279-1284
16. Schroder RJ, Rost B, Hidajat N et al (2002) Value of contrast-enhanced ultrasound vs CT and MRI in palpable enlarged lymph nodes of the head and neck. Rofo Fortschr Geb Rontgenstr neuen Bildgeb Verfahr 174:1099-1106
17. Rubaltelli L, Tregnaghi A, Stramare R (2004) Ultrasonography of superficial lymph nodes: results acquired and new trials. Radiol Med 107:388-346
18. Rubaltelli L, Khadivi Y, Tregnaghi A et al (2004) Evaluation of lymph node perfusion using continuous mode harmonic ultrasonography with a second-generation contrast agent. J Ultrasound Med 23:829-836
19. Schneider M (2000) Design of an ultrasound contrast agent for myocardial perfusion. Echocardiography 17:(Suppl 6 part 2):S11-S16
20. Castelijns JA, van den Brekel MWM (2002) Imaging of lymphadenopathy in the neck. Eur Radiol 12:727-738

Ferdinand Frauscher

Chapter 4

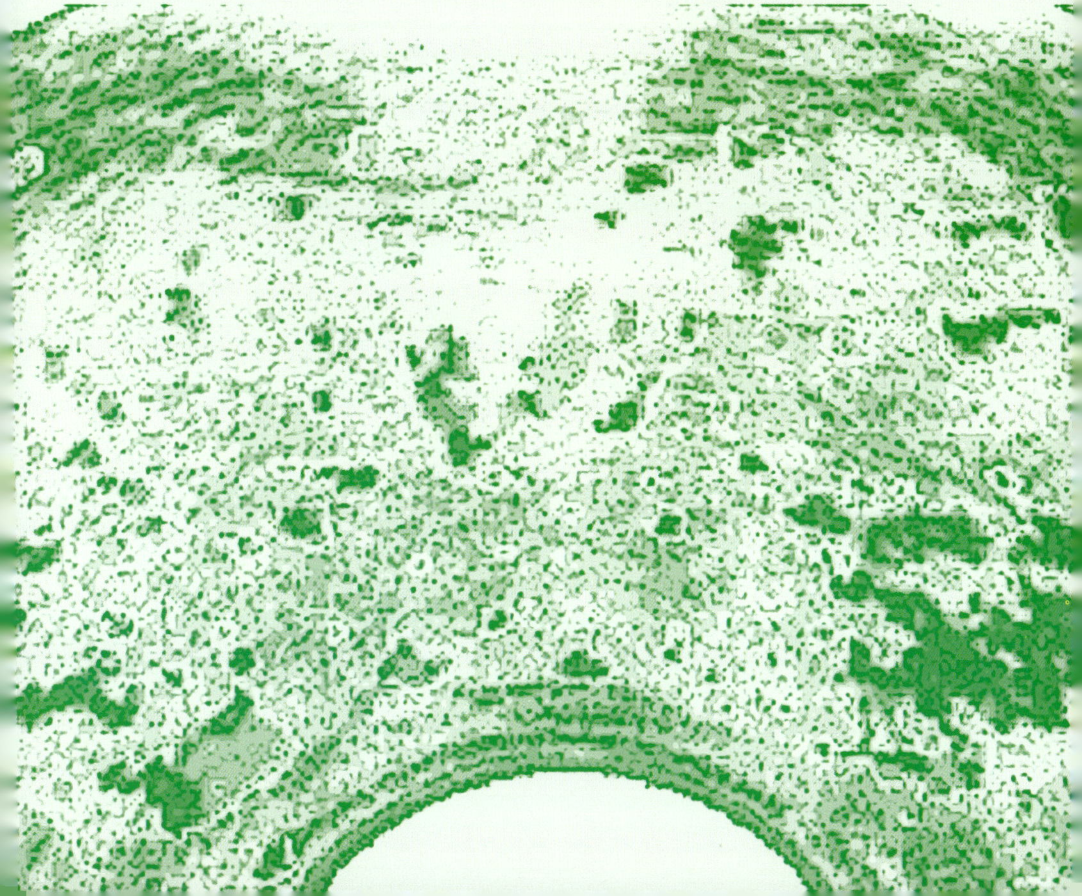

What Role for Contrast-Enhanced Ultrasound in Prostate Cancer Examination?

Ferdinand Frauscher
Department of Radiology, University Hospital Innsbruck, Innsbruck, Austria

Prostate cancer is the most commonly diagnosed malignancy in men. Early diagnosis is essential to provide definitive treatment and improve patient survival. The advent of prostate-specific antigen (PSA) assessment and transrectal ultrasound (US) imaging has revolutionized prostate cancer detection. Gray-scale US has a low sensitivity and specificity for prostate cancer detection. To improve cancer detection, color Doppler imaging (CDI) has been used. Unfortunately, subsequent studies using CDI have reported that CDI misses a considerable number of cancers and is insufficient in avoiding systematic prostate biopsy.

The introduction of US microbubble contrast agents such as SonoVue (Bracco Imaging SpA, Italy) has dramatically expanded the possibilities for US detection of prostate cancer. Several studies have shown that contrast-enhanced CDI (CE-CDI) can improve prostate cancer detection thus reducing the numbers of biopsy cores.

Recent advances in US technology have further increased the value of US contrast agents. Enhanced transrectal gray-scale harmonic US improves the sensitivity for prostate cancer detection without substantial loss of specificity. Contrast-enhanced intermittent US of the prostate seems to be useful for selective enhancement of malignant prostatic tissue. Recent studies evaluating US contrast agent enhancement characteristics (i.e. time intensity curves) reported that this technique provides an objective measure for differentiating benign from malignant prostatic tissue. In summary, these results demonstrate the feasibility of US contrast agents to enhance US imaging of prostatic disease. In our opinion, contrast-enhanced US has the potential to play a major role in the diagnostic evaluation of patients undergoing PSA screening for prostate cancer.

Background

Prostate cancer is the most commonly diagnosed malignancy in men and it is likely to be the most common cause of cancer-related death in men by 2010 [1]. The incidence of prostate cancer is increasing; 24,0000 new cases are estimated in the USA in 2004. Early diagnosis is essential in order to provide definitive treatment and improve patient survival.

The advent of prostate-specific antigen (PSA) assessment and transrectal ultrasound (US) imaging has revolutionized prostate cancer detection [2]. However, although PSA can be assessed with an easy blood test and is very sensitive, it is less specific. As for gray-scale US introduced in the 1980s, it has a good spatial resolution but a low sensitivity and specificity for prostate cancer detection [3], even with high-frequency probes (Fig. 1) and 3D and 4D imaging (Fig. 2). In order to improve cancer detection, color Doppler imaging (CDI) has been used. Unfortunately, subsequent studies have reported that CDI misses a considerable number of cancers and is insufficient in avoiding systematic prostate biopsy [4]. The present diagnostic strategy for the detection of prostate cancer foresees the use of the so-called sextant biopsy which is considered to be the gold standard [5]. However, sextant biopsy may miss clinically detectable prostate cancer in up to 35% of cases. Therefore, new systematic biopsy approaches have been introduced, which utilize laterally directed cores and a higher number of cores [5-8]. However, limitations still exist because, despite the increase in the number of biopsies (up to 18 or more), cancer detection is not increasing [9-11].

Improvement in biopsy techniques is thus necessary and must be attained without increasing the number of biopsy cores, but rather by improving the US imaging technique. Up to now, US has been used to guide the needle for biopsy. We know that an impor-

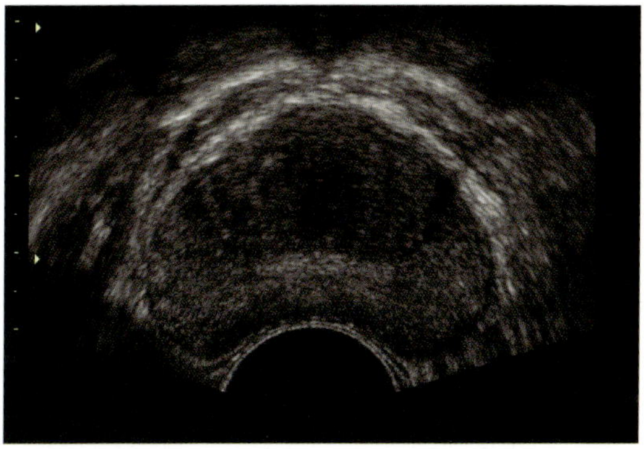

Fig. 1. High-frequency gray-scale US (transverse scan) shows no focal abnormality (i.e., hypoechoic area). Systematic biopsy revealed prostate cancer in the mid right

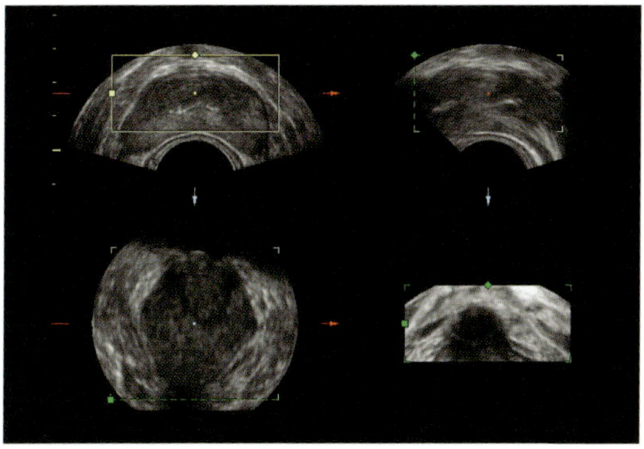

Fig. 2. 3D and 4D gray-scale US images in a patient with prostate cancer in the mid right. No abnormality suggestive of prostate cancer is seen on the US images

tant factor in tumor formation is neoangiogenesis, which through growth factors stimulates new vessel formations, in turn supporting tumor growth. Therefore the detection of neovascularity is crucial for the detection and staging of tumor. However, even with the use of high-end Doppler US systems, a substantial number of cancers can be missed [12]. CDI or power Doppler US is not able to detect lesions that are usually hypovascular and deeply located in the peripheral zone.

The introduction of US microbubble contrast agents has dramatically expanded the possibilities for US detection of prostate cancer [13] as several studies have shown [14-17]. In particular, contrast US applications could allow for new biopsy strategies. In the USA in 2002-2004 the number of biopsies doubled. The introduction of contrast-enhanced ultrasound (CEUS) could be aimed at reducing the number of biopsies necessary to obtain a diagnosis. Moreover, CEUS could help in the staging and grading of prostate cancer, allowing the noninvasive assessment of microvessel density as a prognostic factor. It could also be used in the follow-up after conventional medical (hormonal) and radiation therapy or new therapeutic strategies like high-frequency US (HIFU), radiofrequency ablation, cryotherapy etc.

Our Experience

We used contrast-enhanced CDI with SonoVue (Bracco Imaging, Italy) to detect tumor vascularity in more than 1,500 patients. Results show that prostate cancer was present in 537 of 1,540 subjects (35%) with a mean total PSA level of 3.9 ng/ml. Cancer was detected in 447 subjects (29%) with targeted biopsy, and in 339 of 920 patients (22%) with systematic biopsy.

The percent of cancer detection in targeted biopsies was 13.8%, (997/7,225 cores), while that of systematic biopsies was 5.2% (800/15,400 cores). What is most important in these figures is the huge difference in number of core biopsies necessary for diagnosis, i.e., 7,225 vs 15,400 cores.

Cancers detected with contrast-enhanced targeted biopsy showed a significantly higher Gleason score compared with the systematic technique [16, 17] (Fig. 3). Several studies have also shown that there is a significant correlation between lesion hypervascularity and Gleason score. The Gleason score is a parameter introduced in the 1970s measuring the aggressiveness of tumor. When aggressiveness is high there is a clinically significant cancer and the patient must be treated.

Therefore, contrast-enhanced CDI-targeted biopsy, which detects more prostate cancers with fewer biopsy cores than systematic gray-scale biopsy, can reduce morbidity and costs. Recent advances in US technology, such as harmonic gray-scale imaging with a better temporal resolution, have further increased the value of US contrast agents. Enhanced transrectal gray-scale har-

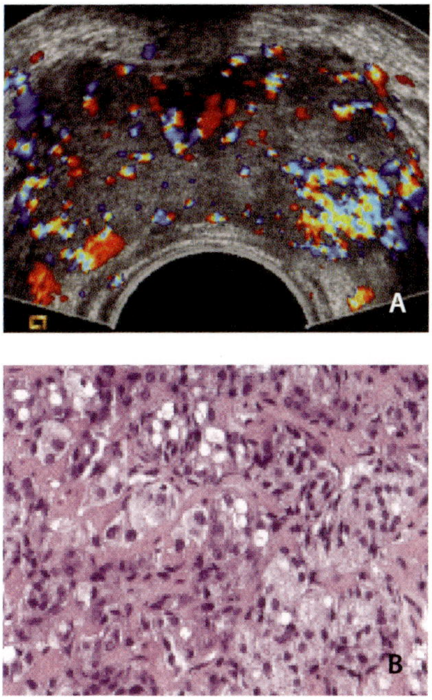

Fig. 3. SonoVue-enhanced color Doppler imaging (CDI) demonstrates hypervascularized area on the left side, which has proven to be a Gleason 9-score cancer. **A** Hypervascularized area on the left side representing prostate cancer. **B** Histology demonstrates Gleason score 9- cancer

monic US improves the sensitivity for prostate cancer detection without substantial loss of specificity [18-20]. Contrast-enhanced intermittent US of the prostate, which reduces the frame rate and allows bubbles to accumulate in the microvessels, seems to be useful for selective enhancement of malignant prostatic tissue [21] (Fig. 4).

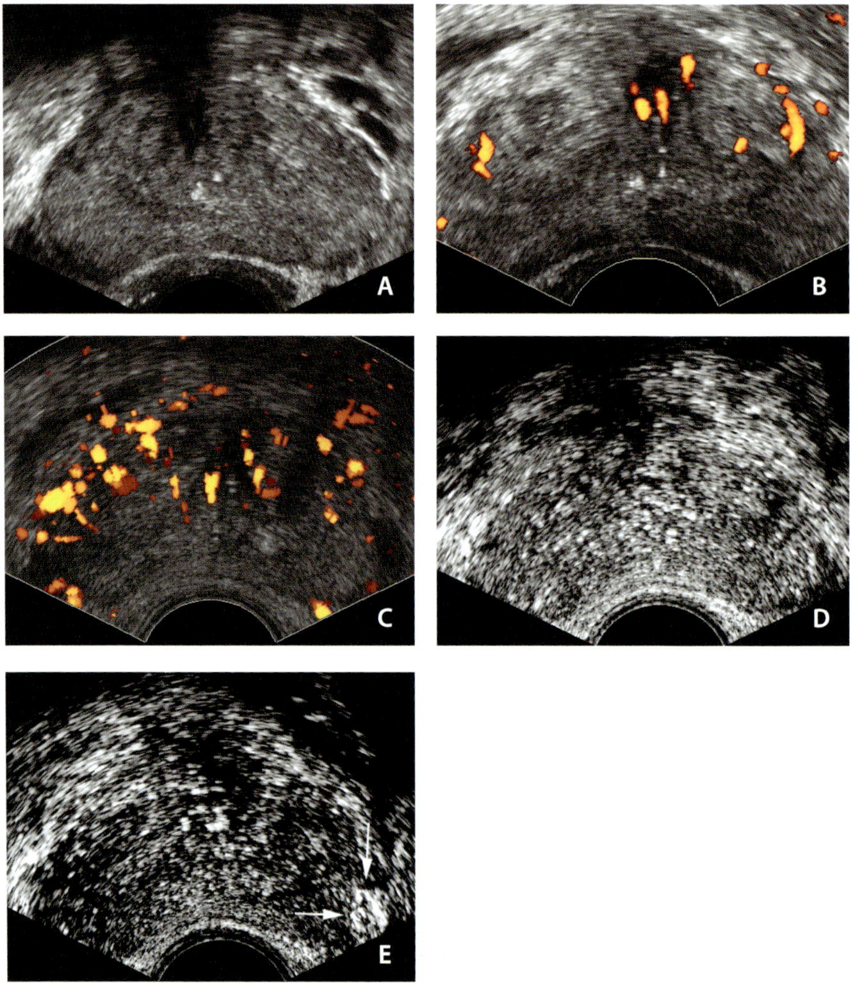

Fig. 4. Prostate cancer: a 55-year-old man with a prostate-specific antigen value of 2.6. **A** - Gray-scale image, no abnormality. **B** Unenhanced power Doppler. No hypervascularized area. **C** Enhanced power Doppler. **D** Continuous gray-scale harmonic US. No suspicious area with enhancement. **E** Intermittent US (delay of 2 s). Enhancing tumor on the left side (*arrows*). Gleason score 7 (4+3)

Preliminary study results with the use of CnTi are also encouraging. Another interesting technique is the assessment of microvessel density. The study of Louvar et al. [22] showed that there is no correlation between conventional color Doppler and microvessel density; however, with the use of contrast agents we showed that this correlation exists (Fig. 5).

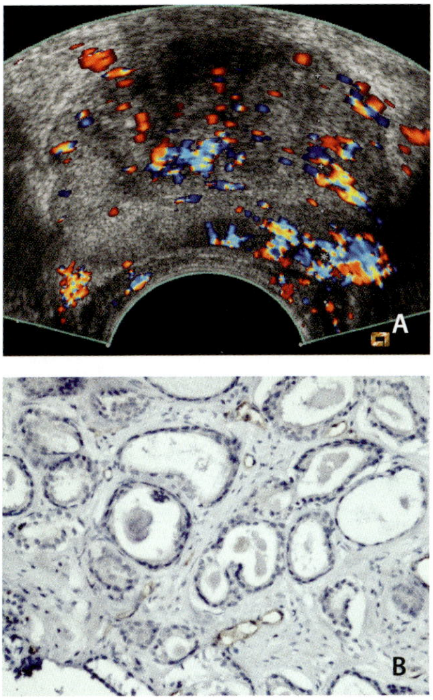

Fig. 5. SonoVue-enhanced CDI shows hypervascularized area on the left, representing prostate cancer. **A** Transversal contrast-enhanced CDI scan. **B** Immunohistochemistry demonstrates high microvessel density (brown outlined vessels)

Another approach is represented by the assessment of the dynamics of contrast agents. Analysis of time of arrival and maximal enhancement demonstrated that it is possible to localize cancer on the basis of time of maximal enhancement.

Recent studies evaluating US contrast agent enhancement characteristics (i.e., time intensity curves) reported that this technique provides an objective measure for differentiating benign from malignant prostatic tissue [23] (Fig. 6). A potential use of contrast agents is also in the follow-up of treatment with hormonal therapy or radiation therapy [24] or to perform local treatment with HIFU [25].

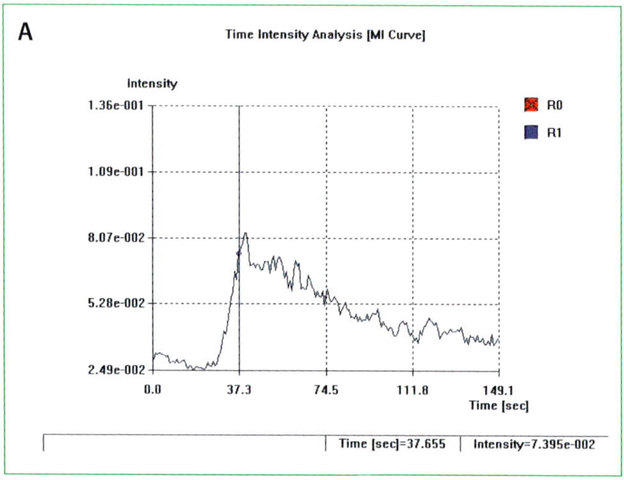

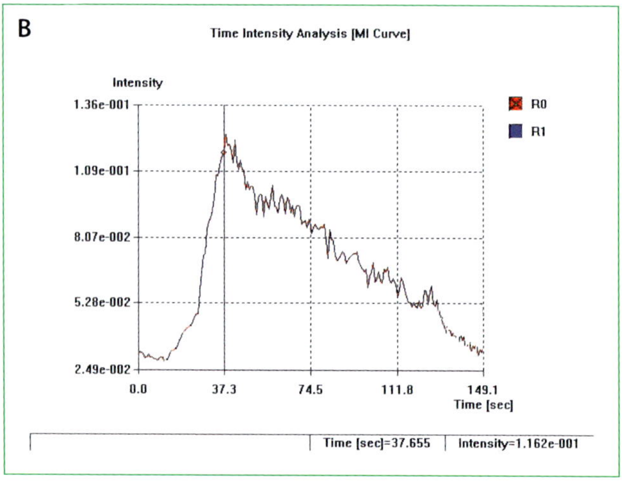

Fig. 6. Time intensity analysis in a patient with prostate cancer of the left side. **A** Contrast agent kinetics obtained from the right side of the prostate without cancer shows lower maximum enhancement. **B** Contrast agent kinetics obtained from the left side of the prostate, wich contains cancer, shows higher maximum enhancement and a faster washout

Conclusion

In summary, these results demonstrate the capability of US contrast agents to enhance US imaging of prostatic disease [26]. The application of US contrast agents for the detection and clinical staging of prostate cancer is promising. Contrast agent-enhanced color Doppler imaging may allow for limited targeted biopsies, thus reducing costs and morbidity. Moreover, it can be useful for treatment follow-up and for the guidance of new therapeutic strategies.

In our opinion, contrast-enhanced US has the potential to play a major role in the diagnostic evaluation of patients undergoing PSA screening for prostate cancer.

References

1. Greenlee RT, Hill-Harmon MB, Murray T, Thun M (2001) Cancer statistics 2001. CA Cancer J Clin 51:15-36
2. Carter HB, Coffey DS (1990) The prostate: an increasing medical problem. Prostate 16:39-48
3. Rifkin MD, Friedland GW, Shortliffe L (1986) Prostatic evaluation by transrectal endosonography: detection of carcinoma. Radiology 158:85-90
4. Halpern EJ, Strup SE (2000) Using gray-scale and color and Power Doppler sonography to detect prostatic cancer. AJR Am J Roentgenol 174:623-627
5. Hodge KK, McNeal JE, Terris MK, Stamey TA (1989) Discussion 74-Random systematic versus directed ultrasound guided transrectal core biopsies of the prostate. J Urol 142:71
6. Stamey TA (1995) Making the most out of six systematic sextant biopsies. Urology 45:2-12
7. Eskew LA, Bare RL, McCullough DL (1997) Systematic 5 region prostate biopsy is superior to sextant method for diagnosing carcinoma of the prostate. J Urol 157:199-202

8. Djavan B, Kadesky K, Klopukh B et al (1998) Gleason scores from prostate biopsies obtained with 18-gauge biopsy needles poorly predict Gleason scores of radical prostatectomy specimens. Eur Urol 33:261-270
9. Naughton CK, Miller DC, Mager DE et al (2000) A prospective randomized trial comparing 6 versus 12 prostate biopsy cores: impact on cancer detection. J Urol 164:388-392
10. Horninger W, Reissigl A, Fink K et al (1998) Results of a prospective randomized study comparing the prostate cancer detection rates in PSA screening volunteers undergoing 10 vs. 14 transrectal ultrasound guided biopsies. J Urol (Suppl)159:180 abstract 690
11. Nava L, Montorsi F, Consonni P et al (1997) Results of a prospective randomised study comparing 6, 12, and 18 transrectal, ultrasound guided, sextant biopsies in patients with elevated PSA, normal DRE and normal prostatic ultrasound. J Urol (Suppl) 15:59 abstract 226
12. Halpern EJ, Frauscher F, Strup SE et al (2002) Prostate: high-frequency Doppler US imaging for cancer detection. Radiology 225:71
13. Goldberg BB, Liu JB, Forsberg F (1994) Ultrasound contrast agents: a review. Ultrasound Med Biol 20:319-333
14. Frauscher F, Helweg G, Gotwald TF et al (1998) The value of contrast-enhanced color Doppler ultrasonography in the diagnosis of prostate cancer. Radiology 209:417
15. Bogers HA, Sedelaar JP, Beerlage HP et al (1999) Contrast-enhanced three-dimensional power Doppler angiography of the human prostate: correlation with biopsy outcome. Urology 54:97-104
16. Frauscher F, Klauser A, Halpern EJ et al (2001) Detection of prostate cancer using a microbubble ultrasound contrast agent. Lancet 357:1849-1851
17. Frauscher F, Klauser A, Volgger H et al (2002) Comparison of contrast enhanced color Doppler targeted biopsy with conventional systematic biopsy: impact on prostate cancer detection. J Urol 167:1648-1652
18. Halpern EJ, Rosenberg M, Gomella LG (2001) Contrast enhanced sonography of the prostate. Radiology 219:219-225

19. Halpern EJ, McCue PA, Aksnes AK et al (2002) Contrast enhanced sonography of the prostate: correlation with whole mount prostatectomy specimens. Radiology 222:361-366
20. Halpern EJ, Frauscher F, Rosenberg M, Gomella LG (2002) Directed biopsy during contrast-enhanced sonography of the prostate. AJR Am J Roentgenol 178:915-919
21. Halpern EJ, Verkh L, Forsberg F et al (2000) Initial experience with contrast-enhanced sonography of the prostate. AJR Am J Roentgenol 174:1575-1580
22. Louvar E, Littrup PJ, Goldstein A et al (1998) Correlation of color Doppler flow in the prostate with tissue microvascularity. Cancer 183:135-140
23. Goossen TE, de la Rosette JJ, Hulsbergen-van de Kaa CA et al (2003) The value of dynamic contrast enhanced ultrasound imaging in the localization of prostate cancer. Eur Urol 43:124-131
24. Eckersley RJ, Sedelaar JP, Blomley MJ et al (2002) Quantitative microbubble enhanced transrectal ultrasound as a tool for monitoring hormonal treatment of prostate carcinoma. Prostate 51:256-267
25. Sedelaar JP, Aarnink RG, van Leenders GJ et al (2000) The application of three-dimensional contrast-enhanced ultrasound to measure volume of affected tissue after HIFU treatment for localized prostate cancer. Eur Urol 37:559-568
26. Frauscher F, Klauser A, Halpern EJ (2002) Advances in ultrasound for the detection of prostate cancer. Ultrasound Q 18:135-142